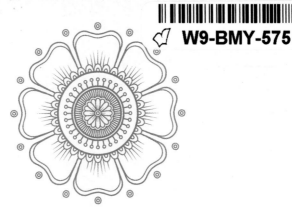

CHINESE

HEALING
SECRETS

pil

Publications International, Ltd.

Cover and interior art: Shutterstock.com

Copyright © 2017 Publications International, Ltd. All rights reserved. This book may not be reproduced or quoted in whole or in part by any means whatsoever without written permission from:

Louis Weber, CEO
Publications International, Ltd.
8140 Lehigh Avenue
Morton Grove, IL 60053

Permission is never granted for commercial purposes.

ISBN: 978-1-68022-710-9

Manufactured in China.

8 7 6 5 4 3 2 1

TABLE OF CONTENTS

INTRODUCTION

As the late afternoon sun sinks behind the mountain, a silent figure walks slowly along the slope. Occasionally he kneels on the ground, gazing at a plant that has caught his attention. After consideration, he digs up some roots and washes them off in a stream. Home is another 15 miles away, in a fertile river valley on the other side of the mountain. Chewing on one of the man-shaped roots, he doesn't seem bothered by the difficult trek that lies ahead of him. After all, he's been taking this trip every autumn for the last 75 years!

When he finally reaches his home village the next morning, children rush up to greet him. When he slides his travel pack off his shoulder, they jump with glee, knowing that he has brought them some treats from the mountains. Reaching into his sack, he hands each child a sweet yellow root. Their mother nods in approval, knowing the roots will ward off the sore throats that are so common with the coming of autumn weather.

Arriving at his hut, he finds villagers waiting. An elderly woman walks up to him, worried that she can't seem to stay warm in the colder weather. Gently holding her wrist, he notices that her pulse is faint and difficult to find. He has already observed that her face and tongue are pale; when she reports that she wakes up throughout the night to urinate, his diagnosis is confirmed. "Not enough yang in the kidneys," he exclaims. He reaches into his medicine bag for a cigar-shaped cylinder of dried herbs and lights it in the communal fire. Gently swirling the smoldering herbs over points below her knees and low back, he instructs an apprentice to prepare an herbal formula for her. The woman is confident that the formula will work—her great-grandmother used the very same herbs when she experienced a similar condition. One by one, the villagers approach the old herbalist, explaining their symptoms to him. In each case, he feels the pulses on both their wrists and looks carefully at their tongue. His diagnoses sound like weather reports: cold and damp; wind with heat; excessive heat leading to dryness. He is a Taoist; his world view consists of an unbroken unity between human beings and the universe that they inhabit.

This perception is at the root of traditional Chinese medicine: The individual (microcosm) is viewed as an integral part of the forces of nature (macrocosm). By careful observation of nature, Taoist sages were able to perceive patterns common to both the external environment and the internal climate of the human body. Over a period of thousands of years, the observations of sages all over China led to an intricate system of diagnosis and healing. The remarkable system of traditional Chinese medicine is one of China's great gifts to humanity. Practically unknown in the West until the 1970s, the secrets of Chinese healing are rapidly becoming part of the mainstream of medicine. The purpose of this book is to share this vast wealth of knowledge and empower you to begin using this ancient wisdom in your own life.

4

THE ROOTS OF TRADITIONAL CHINESE MEDICINE

Archaeological excavations reveal that human beings lived in China more than a million years ago. These primitive people spent most of their time on basic survival: hunting, locating and preparing plants for food, building shelters, and defending themselves. It's easy to imagine that over time, they sampled most of the local plants in their search for food. In time, an oral record evolved that identified those plants that made good food, those that were useful for building, those that had an effect on illness, and those that were poisonous. Through trial and error, a primitive form of herbal medicine and dietary therapy was taking shape in China.

Fire also played a central role in their lives as a source of warmth, fuel, and light. As they huddled around fires, it was only natural that our ancestors would discover the healing powers of heat. Those powers would have been especially evident for cold, damp ailments such as arthritis, for which heat provides immediate relief. This was the origin of the art of moxibustion, the therapeutic application of heat to treat a wide variety of conditions.

These ancient people must have experienced a variety of injuries during their rugged lives. A natural reaction to pain is to rub or press on the affected area. This hands-on therapy gradually evolved into a system of therapeutic manipulation. People discovered that pressing on certain points on the body had wide-ranging effects. They began to use pieces of sharpened bone or stone to enhance the sensation, and acupuncture was born.

WRITTEN HISTORY

The development of a written record of Chinese medicine has evolved mostly over the last 3,000 years. Archeological digs from the Shang Dynasty (1000 BC) have revealed medical writings inscribed on divination bones: Early shamans, mostly women, used scapula bones to perform divination rites; later these bones were also used for writing. The discovery in 1973 of 11 medical texts written on silk has shed some light on the sophisticated practices of that early period of Chinese history. Dated to 168 BC, the texts discuss diet, exercise, moxibustion, and herbal therapy. Liberally mixed with shamanistic magic, an extensive text, *Prescriptions for Fifty-two Ailments*, describes the pharmacologic effects of herbs and foods. Also dating from about this time is the legend of Shen Nong, the Emperor of Agriculture, who tasted 100 herbs daily to assess their qualities. (He is said to have been poisoned many times in the course of his investigations.) The book that is attributed to him is known as the *Classic of the Agriculture Emperor's Materia Medica*. It lists 365 medicines, comprising 252 plants, 67 animals, and 46 minerals. Tao Hong-Jing, the editor of the version of Shen Nong's materia medica in use today, divided the herbs into three classes. The upper-class herbs are nontoxic tonics that strengthen and nourish the body, the middle-grade herbs are tonics with therapeutic qualities, and the lower grade consists of herbs that treat disease or possess some toxicity.

This classification system gives a glimpse into an important principle in traditional Chinese medicine: It is better to strengthen the body and prevent disease than to fight illness once it has already taken hold. Ignoring preventive health care and waiting to treat disease was considered as foolish as waiting until you are thirsty to dig a well.

By AD 400, the basic foundations of traditional Chinese medicine had been put into written form. By this time, most of the magical aspects of medicine had been left behind; there was an increasing belief in the powers of nature to heal disease. The most important book compiled between 300 BC and AD 400 is *The Yellow Emperor's Inner Classic (Huang Di Nei Jing)*. The work is purported to be a series of conversations between the Yellow Emperor, Huang Di, and his minister, Qi Bo, although many historians believe it is a compilation of all the medical knowledge of that period. The work is divided into two books: *Simple Questions and Spiritual Axis*. The first book deals with general theoretical principles, while the second more specifically describes the principles of acupuncture and the treatment of disease.

Remarkably, this ancient work is still valid; it forms the foundation for the contemporary practice of traditional Chinese medicine. For example, the Nei Jing states that cold diseases should be treated with hot herbs, and hot diseases should be treated with cold herbs. This principle is still followed today in clinical practice. Hot, inflammatory infections are treated with cold herbs such as honeysuckle flowers; cold, debilitating conditions such as chronic fatigue are treated with warm, stimulating herbs such as certain kinds of ginseng. Modern research has confirmed that these plants contain constituents with strong pharmacologic effects on these specific conditions.

By the second century AD, physicians all over China were compiling writings of the latest discoveries in acupuncture and herbal medicine. It was during this time that the famous physician Hua Tuo wrote about herbal anesthesia. Although his formula for the anesthetic has been lost, his unique system of acupuncture points is still in use. He was also a pioneer in recommending exercise as a method of maintaining wellness. He is quoted as saying "a running stream never goes bad," meaning exercise moves qi and prevents the stagnation that leads to disease. Another pioneer of the time was Zhang Zhongjing, who wrote *Treatise on Febrile and Miscellaneous Diseases* after witnessing an epidemic that ravaged his city and killed most of his relatives. This highly regarded physician developed a system of diagnosis so sophisticated that it is used by practitioners in modern hospitals 1,700 years after his death.

Between the second and fifth centuries (AD), China experienced a period marked by war and political turmoil. One of the ironies of war is that it has a tendency to lead to advances in medicine. The periodic times of unrest in Chinese history, such as this, were no exception, as the increased need for practical, convenient, effective remedies led to further developments in medical treatment. During this time, Ge Hong wrote *Prescriptions for Emergencies* in order to spread the knowledge of acupuncture and moxibustion to the masses. Around AD 650, Sun Simiao compiled *Prescriptions Worth A Thousand Gold*, which integrated the clinical experiences of the different schools of acupuncture at that time. During the Tang Dynasty (618–907), China's Imperial Medical Bureau established departments of Acupuncture, Pharmacology, and Medical Specialties, and numerous additional treatises and compilations of medical knowledge and experience were prepared.

In the Five Dynasties period (907–1368), advancements in printing techniques led to a dramatic increase in the publication of medical texts. One of the important books of the period was *Canon on the Origin of Acupuncture and Moxibustion,* in which Wang Zhizhong incorporated the clinical experiences of the practitioners of folk medicine. During the Ming Dynasty (1368–1644), many medical specialists compiled the works of their forebears, further expanding the extensive base of medical knowledge. The most famous physician of the period was Li Shi Zheng (1518–1593), a kind and generous healer who did not accept payment for his services. After reviving the son of a prince from a coma, he was appointed court physician and served in the Imperial Academy of Medicine. His most incredible achievement was his 40-year effort in writing the *Ben Cao Gong Mu (General Catalog of Herbs),* a monumental work published after his death. Consisting of 52 volumes at the time of its printing, the *Ben Cao Gong Mu* remains an important reference for traditional Chinese herbalists.

RECENT HISTORY

The integration of new techniques with ancient understanding continued up until the time of the Opium War of 1840. This catastrophic event turned China into a semi-colonial society. Western colonial powers derided traditional medicine as primitive and outdated. When the Communist party came to power in the middle of the twentieth century, they brought much turmoil to China; however, the Communists saw the need to promote traditional Chinese medicine to avoid dependence on the West. A great need for traditional doctors arose since there were far too few Western-trained physicians to serve the huge population: only 10,000 Western-trained doctors were available to serve 400 million people. Traditional Chinese medicine began a course of revival that continues today.

Many Western-trained physicians and scientists in China started to conduct research on acupuncture, moxibustion, and herbal medicine, and a gradual integration of the two systems began. In 1945, an acupuncture clinic opened in a Western hospital in China for the first time.

Since then, traditional Chinese medicine and Western medicine have been practiced side by side in Chinese hospitals, sometimes by a physician who has been trained in both fields. For example, a cancer patient might receive radiation to treat a tumor then be sent to the herbal department for formulas to strengthen his immune system and normalize his blood count.

Since the 1970s, Chinese hospitals have trained students from more than 100 countries in the principles of traditional medicine. Interest in traditional Chinese medicine was sparked in the United States in the early 1970s when *The New York Times* reporter James Reston experienced an acute appendicitis attack while in China. His report of receiving acupuncture to relieve his postoperative abdominal pain brought an awareness of this system of healing to the general public. Since then, acupuncture and herbal medicine have gradually taken hold in North America. With more than 10,000 practitioners and an increasing number of schools of traditional Chinese medicine, this ancient system has taken its well-deserved place in the Western world.

YIN AND YANG

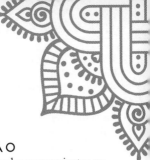

BEGIN WITH THE TAO

Although there are many definitions of Tao, this one word communicates an entire philosophy, an outlook on the fundamental nature of life and the universe. The word Tao is nothing less than an expression of the profound unity of the universe and of the path human beings must take to join, rather than disturb, that unity.

What is this path, and how do we find it? The path begins with an understanding of the origin of the universe. "Knowing the ancient beginning is the essence of the way," stated the ancient Chinese sage Lao Tzu, the author of the *Tao Te Ching*. Known in English as *The Book of the Way*, this poetic masterpiece was written approximately 2,500 years ago. As well as being a matchless work of literature, it takes its place in history as the first written record of Taoist philosophy.

THE STORY OF CREATION

The Taoist theory of creation is not unlike other traditional creation stories. At first, there was simply a great void, the ultimate quiescence, called "Wu Chi." Wu Chi is also understood as creative potential, primal force, and universal energy. Wu Chi, the source, created the two opposites: yang, the active force, and yin, the passive force. These two forces are perpetually changing, one into the other; their interplay gives birth to the transformation of matter, called "the 10,000 things"—the Taoist expression for everything in the universe. When the perfect balance between yin and yang is achieved, there is harmony, epitomized by the Tai Chi (yin-yang) symbol. Tao is found first by encompassing, and then by balancing, the extremes of both polarities.

Lao Tzu's *Tao Te Ching*, an extraordinary work of 81 mysterious and beautiful verses, offers council for wounded hearts, a path for the lost, and a balm for troubled brows. This compendium of Taoist thought begins:

The Tao that can be told
is not the true Tao.
The name that can be named
is not the eternal name.
The nameless is the beginning of heaven and earth.
The named is the mother

9

of the ten thousand things.
Ever desireless,
one can see the mystery.
Ever desiring, one can see
the manifestations.
These two spring from the same source but differ in name;
this appears as darkness.
Darkness within darkness.
The gate to all mystery.

Enigmatic and mystical, like all Taoist poetry, this first verse unveils the Taoist understanding of creation and the mystical path of the Tao. It tells us that about Wu Chi, the ultimate void, the eternal, we can say nothing. Its depths are beyond our reaches. We can only reflect on its manifestations: the yin and yang and all that these two forces create; that is, the world we live in and all that is in it. But the study of the interplay between these two forces is enough to start us on the path. By seeking harmony within ourselves, and between ourselves and the outside world and all its inhabitants, we will be able to achieve a superior state of being. By existing in this state of perpetual balance, we develop a true perspective on the nature of life and its unseen source.

Whoever achieves this state achieves "teh," often translated as virtue in the sense of perfection. The person who does not seek to live in harmony with the Tao will remain lopsided with desire, never being able to see things as they are and never comprehending more than what the physical world offers. Lao Tzu makes it clear from the outset that when we search for Tao, we do so without the tools of intellect and language. Using these tools would put the Tao forever beyond our grasp. So it is on the strength of our natural intuitions, guided by the images of poets and painters, that we walk the path, speechlessly seeking Tao, the inexpressible.

Through patient observation of the forces of nature, the Taoists who developed the system of traditional Chinese medicine saw the universe as a unified field, constantly moving and changing while maintaining its oneness. They used the theory of the yin and the yang to explain this constant state of change.

They believed nature expresses itself in an endless cycle of polar opposites such as day and night, moisture and dryness, heat and cold, and activity and rest. Yin phenomena are those that exhibit the nurturing qualities of darkness, rest, moisture, cold, and structure. Its Chinese character depicts the shady side of a hill. Yang phenomena have qualities of energy such as light, activity, dryness, heat, and function. Its Chinese character represents the sunny side of a hill.

Everything in nature exhibits varying combinations of both yin and yang. For example, the morning fog (yin) is dissipated by the heat of the sun (yang); the forest fire (yang) is extinguished by the rainstorm (yin); the darkness of night (yin) is replaced by the light of day (yang). Any phenomenon within nature can be understood in relation to another; one will always be yin or yang in comparison with the other.

Some of the basic principles of yin and yang:

- Everything in nature can be expressed as the opposition of yin and yang. This is the energizing force of all aspects of nature. It is dynamic and the basic foundation for change in nature. Yin and yang are also relative terms: A forest fire is more yang than a campfire; a campfire is more yang than a spark. Nothing is purely yin or yang; it is always a matter of comparison.

- Yin and yang are interdependent. Even though yin and yang are opposites, one has no meaning without the other. For example, day would have no meaning without night; heat cannot be understood without knowing what cold feels like; fever and chills can't be determined without experiencing the normal body temperature.

- Yin creates yang; yang creates yin. Numerous examples of this principle can be seen in nature. For example, on a hot summer day (yang), there is a sudden thunderstorm (yin). A person may get symptoms of chills and a runny nose (yin) that turn into a fever with a sore throat (yang). A hyperactive child runs around frantically (yang), then suddenly falls asleep (yin).

- Yin and yang mutually control each other. This is the basic mechanism of balance in nature and the human body. When the body gets overheated from exercise, the pores open and sweating lowers the temperature. When the body gets too cold due to exposure, the muscles shiver to generate heat.

Since the Taoists believe that everything is part of the oneness of the universe, they do not make a distinction between the external forces of nature and the internal processes of the human body, believing that "the macrocosm exists within the microcosm." In other words, any process or change that can be witnessed in nature can also be observed in the body. For example, a person who eats cold food (yin) on a cold, damp day (yin) may experience excessive mucus (yin). Similarly, a person who performs strenuous activity (yang) on a hot day (yang) might experience dehydration along with a fever (yang). Some of the traditional diagnoses sound like weather reports, such as "wind and cold with dampness" (a yin condition) or a "deficiency of moisture leading to fire" (a yang pattern). These diagnostic descriptions illustrate the principle that the human body experiences the same fluctuations of yin and yang as the external environment.

The internal organs also have their own balance of yin and yang. Yin functions tend to be nourishing, cooling, building, and relaxing, and relate to the structure, or substance, of the organs. Yang qualities tend to be energizing, warming, consuming, and stimulating and relate to the functional activity of the organs. For example, the kidneys are considered the source of yin (water) and yang (fire, or metabolism) for the entire body. If the kidney yin is deficient or depleted, a person can experience hot flashes and night sweats, as occurs in menopause when estrogen (yin) levels decline. This is due to insufficient moisture (yin) to keep the metabolic fire (yang), which keeps the body warm, under control. Think of running a car engine with insufficient oil; the engine will overheat due to a deficiency of this yin-like lubricant. A deficiency of kidney yang produces such symptoms as cold hands and feet and a general lack of vitality. These symptoms, which often occur with age, are due to insufficient metabolic fire (yang) to infuse the entire body with energy and warmth, dispersing cold and fatigue (yin).

Traditional Chinese medicine applies this ancient theory of yin and yang in clinical practice. In the case of kidney yin deficiency, the therapeutic principle is to tonify (fortify) the yin and sedate the hyperactive yang. This is achieved with a classic formula known as "Rehmannia Teapills," which contain three herbs that nourish the kidneys' yin and three herbs that clear the heat that arises from the lack of the cooling and moistening yin functions. In kidney yang deficiency, similar herbs are used to nourish the kidney, with the addition of warming metabolic stimulants such as aconite root and cinnamon bark. Since all the organs have similar yin and yang aspects, it is possible to monitor and adjust the yin and yang levels of all parts of the body, maintaining a high level of vitality and preventing disease. This is achieved not only with herbs but with changes in diet and lifestyle. In this way, the ancient observations of the Taoists have practical applications in our own quest for wellness.

THE VITAL
SUBSTANCES

In traditional Chinese medicine, the body and mind are inseparable. Composed of a number of vital substances—qi (pronounced chee), blood, essence, and body fluids—the body and mind express their qualities through the functions of the internal organs. Ranging from tangible, visible substances to subtle, intangible ones, these elements of the body/mind are responsible for all aspects of human life—physical, mental, emotional, and spiritual. Their intimate involvement in human activity makes them an essential part of physiology, and recognition and understanding of them are an essential part of diagnosis.

Q I

The idea of qi is not easily accepted by Westerners. It is not a concept that appears in our mainstream religions or philosophies. Neither do our medical and scientific traditions acknowledge qi or even have any place for it in their theories. In China and the Orient, however, the concept of qi is very familiar, even commonplace. Everyone, from politicians to school children, understands it. The notion of qi and its applications are as much a part of Chinese life and outlook as are the ideas of muscle tone and physical fitness in Western life.

Easterners believe qi to be the life energy contained within matter. In experiments conducted in the 1960s, nuclear physicists in China came to accept the notion that it is actually a low-frequency, highly concentrated form of infrared radiation. In the last decade, experiments in China have been conducted on this special type of energy. Some researchers have come to believe, just as the legends tell us, that certain people may be able to learn to emit this form of energy from their bodies. These highly trained individuals often devote their lives to developing this subtle energy.

Although qi plays a central role in traditional Chinese medicine, it is extremely difficult to define. It is best to understand it in terms of its functions and activities, where it is more readily perceived. Situated somewhere between matter and energy, qi has the qualities of both. It has substance without structure, and it possesses energy qualities but can't be measured. It is the fundamental power underlying all the activities of nature as well as the vital life force of the human body. For example, the force of a thunderstorm can be understood in terms of its qi: The power of qi can be observed in the fallen trees and buildings in the storm's aftermath. Similarly, the strength of the digestive organs can be determined in relation to their qi by evaluating the appetite, color of the tongue, strength of the pulse, and the body's response to nutrition.

Most people are understandably skeptical about this energy until they actually experience it for themselves. After all, in the West we have been well trained to deny even the possibility of such phenomena. While some people will never be able to sense the qi, many others do—some on their first encounter with it.

Try this experiment with a partner, such as your child, spouse, or friend, to see if you are able to feel the qi. Both of you should either sit or stand approximately two arm-lengths away from each other. Ask your partner to close his eyes and take a deep breath. Relax your shoulders and back muscles as completely as possible. Try to imagine an energy rising from the ground into your body.

When you think you can almost sense this imaginary force, ask your partner to extend an arm toward you until it is level with the floor. The palm of the hand should be facing downward. Slowly raise your own arms and extend your fingers until they are within a few inches of your partner's outstretched hand. Using your mind, direct the imaginary energy—what we call the qi. Move it further up through your body until it passes along your arms and out from your fingertips. It's helpful to imagine a current of energy passing from your body into your partner's. Whether you think this is an imaginary force or not, some people feel the qi right away, even with their eyes closed.

More powerful demonstrations of the application of qi can be found in Chinese medical centers, where acupuncture techniques are used on patients ready to undergo surgery. The acupuncture is used to stimulate the qi, which then induces anesthesia. Using these techniques, patients regularly undergo major operations without drugs.

The flow of qi through the body occurs within a closed system of channels, or meridians. There are 12 major meridians, and they correspond to the 12 organ systems: six yin organs and six yang organs. Traditional organ theory pairs yin and yang organs according to their structure and function and the interconnection of their meridians. In addition, eight extra meridians are interconnected with all the channels. This network of meridians allows the qi, or life force, to reach all the tissues and organs, providing nourishment, warmth, and energy to all parts of the body. The flow of qi travels from channel to channel, passing through all the meridians every 24 hours. For example, the flow of qi in the heart meridian is strongest between the hours of 11 a.m. and 1 p.m. From there, the qi flows into the meridian of the small intestine, staying there until 3 p.m., at which time the flow passes into the bladder meridian. In this way, qi passes through all the major meridians and their corresponding organs every day. Although the meridians are deep within the body, points along them are accessible from the surface of the skin. It is the manipulation of these points by means of pressure, heat, or needles that is the basis for acupressure, moxibustion, and acupuncture, respectively. The qi that flows through the meridians can be manipulated at the acupuncture points, bringing healing energy to organs that need it and moving energy away from areas that are impaired due to stagnation of qi.

FUNCTIONS OF QI

Although many types of specialized qi exist in the body, such as those associated with a particular organ, all varieties share some basic functions. These functions are as follows:

- Transformation: Qi transforms one type of substance into another. Spleen qi transforms food into qi and blood the body can use; kidney qi transforms fluids into pure essence and waste water; lung qi transforms air into the energy to sustain life.

- Movement: All movement is accompanied by its own qi, including growth and development and even walking, breathing, and thinking. Qi moves the blood through the vessels, giving rise to the saying, "Qi is the commander of the blood."

- Protection: Qi protects the body from attacks by disease-causing organisms. Therefore, if a person's qi is weak, that person may experience frequent illnesses.

- Retention: Qi keeps the organs in their proper place, keeps blood within the vessels, and keeps body fluids inside the body. Deficiency of qi can lead to sagging organs (prolapse), bleeding disorders, and excessive sweating or urination.

- Warming: The yang aspect of kidney qi keeps the entire body warm; when it is deficient, chronic cold extremities and decreased function in all activities that require warmth, such as digestion, can occur.

TYPES OF QI

Chinese medicine traditionally divides qi into various types, depending on its source and function. The original source of this life force is a person's parents, and the qi inherited from them is known as prenatal qi. Prenatal qi, the basic constitution of a human being, depends on genetics and the quality of the parents' lives at the time of conception and during pregnancy. This qi initially locates in and around the kidneys. As the organs of the body begin to function autonomously, the prenatal qi moves into the rest of the body. This qi is the person's heritage, and it cannot be replenished; however, healthy lifestyle, diet, and breathing practices can conserve prenatal qi and slow down its depletion. Preservation of prenatal qi is one of the most important contributions of traditional Chinese medicine. It enables a person who is sickly and weak to live a life of health and vitality. The process involves a simultaneous conservation of prenatal qi with practices that enhance the formation of postnatal qi.

Postnatal qi, or acquired qi, is derived from the digestion of food and extracted from the air we breathe. Combined with prenatal qi, it forms the totality of the body's power to perform all the vital processes of life. One of the functions of the lungs is to extract qi from air and incorporate it into the storehouse of postnatal qi. The strength of postnatal qi depends on a number of factors: the strength of lung qi, the quality of the air, and the performance of breathing exercises such as qi gong, which enhances the lungs' ability to extract qi from air. When lung qi is deficient, a person can experience symptoms of fatigue, shortness of breath, pallor, and frequent colds. The other factor in building strong postnatal qi is the quality of the food we eat and the strength of our digestive organs, especially the spleen. When spleen qi is weak, symptoms of fatigue, lack of appetite, sluggishness, and loose stools can occur. When the diet lacks essential nutrients and variety, the extraction of qi is impaired even if spleen qi is strong. People accustomed to eating fresh organic fruits, vegetables, and whole grains will often experience this when circumstances force them to eat denatured, refined, pesticide-laden foods: Inevitably, they notice their energy level drops. Recent research has confirmed that organically grown produce has significantly higher levels of nutrients.

When both spleen qi and lung qi are strong, and the quality of our air and food are high, postnatal qi can grow. Herbs that tonify lung and spleen qi, along with breathing practices such as qi gong, further increase the accumulation of postnatal qi. In this way, even a person with a weak inherited constitution (prenatal qi) can experience a life of health and vitality.

The totality of qi that results from the combination of prenatal and postnatal qi is known as true qi. Responsible for all the functions of the body, true qi takes different forms. From the clinical perspective, two of these forms of qi are especially significant: nutritive qi and protective qi.

Nutritive qi circulates in the meridians and nourishes the organs. Acupuncture manipulates this qi to affect organ function. Specific points along the meridians are needled, pressed, or warmed (by means of moxibustion) to achieve specific effects in the organs. For example, a point below the knee is manipulated traditionally to treat appendicitis, often eliminating the symptoms when the condition is caught before infection sets in. When a Chinese surgeon performing appendectomies needled this point on his patients, he found that the intestines contracted rhythmically on either side of the appendix. This demonstrates how the power of qi can be observed, even when it is difficult to understand exactly how it is working.

The other important subdivision of true qi is protective qi, or wei qi. Believed to flow between the skin and muscles, wei qi is responsible for defending the body from external pathogens that attack the body. Although first described thousands of years ago, wei qi accurately describes the body's immune system. Research has confirmed that herbs traditionally used to tonify wei qi, such as *Astragalus* root (huang qi), have a powerful effect in strengthening the body's resistance to disease and increasing immune function.

SEEING IS BELIEVING

One simple but very convincing feat that demonstrates the power and presence of qi is known as "weight underside." This demonstration does not rely on physical strength, so even those who are relatively small in stature but familiar with the technique can give a very convincing performance. Two strong men stand on either side of the practitioner, each holding one arm, which is bent at the elbow and parallel to the floor. The bend in the arm makes a convenient supporting frame so the men have excellent leverage. Try as they might, after the initial preparation, the men will not be able to move the master, no matter how much force they use. It quickly becomes a comical sight—two burly fellows looking desperate and shifting positions in a hopeless effort to move one average-size person from the standing position.

Such a feat cannot be accomplished without special knowledge of qi. The secret is using the mind to direct the qi, which is used to "move" body weight to an imaginary location somewhere beneath the surface of the floor. As a result, the practitioner becomes virtually immovable. Once the central concepts are learned, masters say the exercise is quite easy to accomplish with regular practice. Using the mind to direct the qi is one of the central ideas in many of the martial arts. By training the mind in this way, practitioners can perform many astounding feats.

Weight underside is only one of many applications for qi. Other convincing demonstrations of the power of qi are related not only to combat but also to the healing arts. Qi is commonly used to relieve pain and stiffness of limbs and joints, to induce sleep, and to promote the healing of damaged organs or other body tissues. Advanced practitioners believe that when the qi circulates freely through the body, it can awaken latent psychic abilities. Some are able to absorb qi from the world around them and later emit it as a powerful radiation. Demonstrations of the power of qi are often given at various gatherings in Chinese communities.

DISORDERS OF QI

Chinese medicine seeks to ensure that the levels, direction, and flow of qi are all appropriate for their particular organs. The various disorders of qi that can occur involve deficiency, sinking, stagnation, or incorrect movement of qi.

The symptoms of qi deficiency are common to all the types of qi disorders: fatigue, pallor, and lethargy. When the qi of an organ is deficient, the specific functions of that organ are also impaired. For example, the spleen is responsible for appetite and digestion; spleen qi deficiency produces poor appetite and loose stools. Lung qi is responsible for the strength of respiration; when it is deficient, a person experiences shortness of breath and a chronic cough. In disorders of sinking qi, the qi that holds organs in place has insufficient strength to do its job. The result is sagging, prolapsed organs, such as the uterus, transverse colon, or rectum. Specific acupuncture points and herbs can correct this type of imbalance.

When qi is stagnant, the functions of an organ are impaired due to a blockage in its qi flow. The liver is the organ most often affected. Since the liver is in charge of the smooth flow of emotion, stagnant liver qi frequently results in irritability. Because there is sufficient qi, tonifying in these cases would make the situation worse, so treatment focuses on moving qi away from the area.

In rebellious qi, the normal direction of organ qi is reversed. Each organ has a normal direction of qi flow; for example, the lungs and stomach move qi downward, while the spleen moves qi upward. Rebellious lung qi results in coughing or wheezing; rebellious stomach qi produces symptoms of nausea, belching, or vomiting; and rebellious spleen qi produces diarrhea.

BLOOD

In traditional Chinese medicine, blood has parallels to its Western counterpart, such as its function of circulating through the body and nourishing the organs. However, it also has some very subtle functions in traditional Chinese medicine, such as providing a foundation for the mind and improving sensitivity of the sensory organs. In other words, a deficiency of blood causes an impairment in mental function, leading to poor memory, anxiety, and insomnia. Blood deficiency can also impair the senses, especially the eyes, causing blurry vision. Closely aligned with qi, blood has a complementary relationship with it. The saying, "Blood is the mother of qi, and qi is the leader of blood," refers to the fact that without blood, qi has no fundamental nutritional basis; without qi, the body cannot form or circulate blood, and the blood would fail to stay within the vessels. The two are considered to flow together through the body.

DISORDERS OF BLOOD

Blood's main function is to circulate throughout the body, providing nourishment and moisture to the organs, skin, muscles, and tendons. When it is deficient, symptoms such as dry skin, inflexible tendons, and various emotional and reproductive imbalances can occur, depending on the organs involved. Since qi and blood are so closely related, a deficiency or stagnation of one of the substances often leads to the same type of imbalance in the other one.

The organs that have the most intimate relationship with blood are the spleen, heart, and liver. The spleen creates qi and blood from food; it also helps keep blood within the vessels. When spleen qi is deficient, blood deficiency or bleeding disorders can occur. The heart is said to "rule the blood and vessels." When it is qi or yang deficient, energy to move blood through the vessels is insufficient, resulting in poor circulation and feelings of coldness in the extremities. Since the heart blood is also the resting place for the mind and spirit, deficient heart blood leads to symptoms of insomnia, palpitations, restlessness, and poor memory. Finally, the liver stores the blood during times of rest or sleep. This function is a process of regeneration, and it is also intimately involved with menstrual flow and fertility. A deficiency of liver blood can lead to scanty menstruation or infertility. Stagnant liver blood may lead to menstrual cramping and discomfort. Since the liver opens into the eyes, this deficiency can also produce such symptoms as blurry vision, floaters, and dry eyes.

BODY FLUIDS

Body fluids refer to all the fluids in the body, such as sweat, tears, saliva, and various secretions and lubricants. The spleen and stomach regulate the formation of fluids, which are considered byproducts of digestion, while the intestines and bladder are involved in their excretion. The lungs regulate body fluids from above, and the kidneys are in charge of their metabolism throughout the body. Fluids consist of two basic types: clear thin fluids known as jin, and thick viscous fluids known as ye. Jin is distributed mostly to the muscles and skin, keeping them moist and nourished. Ye acts as a lubricant to the joints and nourishes the brain. Jin ye is the collective term for all the body fluids.

Because of the relationship between the organs and body fluids, a traditional Chinese medicine practitioner can extrapolate a wealth of information about organ function from the condition of the jin ye. For this reason, the initial interview includes questions about thirst, urination, color of fluids, and the amount and timing of sweating. Sweat is ruled by the heart. Excessive sweating during the day is considered a sign of yang deficiency; night sweats, on the other hand, are a sign of yin deficiency. Tears relate to the liver; dry eyes are a sign of liver blood and yin deficiency. Sputum is ruled by the spleen; excessive sputum is a symptom of yin excess in the spleen. The lungs are the storage area for mucus; a runny nose or wet cough is a sign of yin excess in the lungs. Since the kidneys control the moisture of the entire body, a dry mouth can indicate kidney yin deficiency.

The body fluids also have an intimate relationship with qi. Since qi is involved in the transformation of fluids, deficient qi can lead to fluid retention or excessive sweating. Conversely, fluid stagnation can impair qi circulation, and profuse loss of body fluid can lead to a severe deficiency of qi. For this reason, herbs that induce sweating are used cautiously in people who are qi deficient.

QI AND BREATHING

Knowledge of qi is not today, and never has been, exclusive to China. The idea that qi is an "intelligent" energy that protects the body and coordinates its functions has appeared in many cultures. This "living energy" is called prana in India, and in fact it very likely has been studied in that country for a longer period of time than in China itself. In his book *The Hindu-Yogi Science of Breath*, Yogi Ramacharaka succinctly describes prana: "Prana is the name by which we designate a universal principle, which is the essence of all motion force or energy, whether manifested in gravitation, electricity, the revolution of the planets, and all forms of life, from the highest to the lowest. This great principle is in all forms of matter, and yet it is not matter. It is in the air, but it is not air nor one of its chemical constituents. Animal and plant life breathe it in with the air, and yet if they contained it not they would die even though they might be filled with air."

The notion that qi is related to breath was a favorite theme of the Indian sages of the Vedic Period. (Veda means wisdom in Sanskrit, the holy language of ancient India.) During this period, which began nearly four thousand years ago, the ancient sages began to record their ideas in written form. Many texts from the Vedic Period have been preserved to this day. Studying this literature, we realize that the idea of relating qi and breath is as old as recorded history. In Sanskrit, prana means "ultimate energy," and when used in context with living organisms, it is recognized as the "vital animating force" in living things. Ever since that time, practitioners have believed that it was necessary to breathe to acquire this force, so the intimate relationship between the act of breathing and staying alive and well was established in this way. Consequently, innumerable breathing exercises from many different sects were developed specifically to increase the amount of available qi and to use it for special purposes.

Exactly who these ancient sages might have been, no one knows. The only traces of them are found in the Vedic literature and perhaps in some yogic practices. Their legacy, however, offers a wealth of information on topics related to the vital force in human life and how it may be purified. They observed in their incomparably poetic way, for example, that the basic emotions, such as fear, passion, rage, and anxiety, would cause corresponding physiological responses, all negative. The yogis, who later followed these secret teachings, noticed that these physical states were invariably related to, among other things, heart rate, muscular tension, and respiratory rate, and that undesirable mental states, such as confusion and disorientation, accompanied these changes.

Breathing control, as it turned out, was central to their success in regulating these physiological responses. By controlling such variables as the volume of air, the rate at which it is inhaled and exhaled, the timing between the inhale and exhale, and the location in the lungs in which the air is placed, they could affect both mental and physical states of being. Using carefully prescribed breathing patterns, the masters learned to induce special states, such as deep meditation or heightened awareness, for use in specific situations. As a result of their painstaking research over the course of centuries, the masters made exciting discoveries related to health, strength, longevity, and even happiness. These ideas were systematized and became a basic part of the many different systems of psycho-physical exercises such as yoga. It was during this period of research that the relationship between breath and qi was firmly established.

It seems there is considerable truth to the hypothesis that special breathing techniques can indeed enhance certain functions of the body. It is well known, for example, that children with weak respiratory systems may be able to overcome their deficiencies if given a wind instrument to practice at a young age. The idea is that the act of exercising the lungs consistently over long periods of time will strengthen the muscle groups responsible for respiratory functions and increase the supply of oxygen to the entire body. According to traditional Chinese medical theory, by strengthening their breathing, children will increase the quantity of available pectoral qi, which is not only responsible for respiratory functions but also for the proper operation of the heart.

ESSENCE AND SPIRIT

Stored in the kidneys, essence (jing) is the subtle substance that is responsible for growth, development, and reproduction. Prenatal essence is inherited from the parents, and it is the original substance of life. It cannot be increased, but it can be conserved through a healthy lifestyle and moderation. It can be supplemented with postnatal essence, which is derived from nutrition. When the essence is strong, a child grows and develops normally and enjoys healthy brain function and strong immunity and fertility as an adult. Conversely, birth defects, mental retardation, and a child's failure to thrive are considered signs of a deficiency of essence. In adults, essence deficiency can cause infertility, low immunity, and premature aging.

Spirit (shen) is a person's innate vitality. It can be considered the soul, but it also has a material aspect. When an individual has healthy shen, the eyes have the glow of life and the mind is clear. Since the heart is the resting place for the spirit, disturbances in shen are typically diagnosed as heart imbalances. A mild shen syndrome appears with a heart blood deficiency, with signs of forgetfulness, insomnia, fatigue, and restlessness. In a more serious shen syndrome, "heat phlegm confusing the heart," the individual may be violent, with red face and eyes; the Western diagnosis of this condition might be psychosis. A person who is in a coma as a result of a stroke or a person who experiences epileptic seizures may receive a diagnosis of the shen disturbance known as "phlegm blocking the heart opening."

THE INTERNAL ORGANS

The understanding and description of the internal organ structures and systems in traditional Chinese medicine is remarkably sophisticated, considering the fact that traditional organ theory was developed between 559 and 479 BC. It was considered a violation of the sanctity of life to perform dissections, so organ theory was developed on the basis of how the body functions. The body was viewed holistically, with the understanding that all functions necessary to maintain health were innately present within its internal organs. By means of careful observation, the Taoists were able to see functional relationships among seemingly unrelated activities, actions, emotions, and sensory perceptions.

The function and structure of the vital organs in traditional Chinese medicine differ from that of similarly named organs in Western medicine. It's true that in some cases, the functional relationships closely parallel those established in Western medicine. For example, the Taoists reasoned that "the kidneys govern water." Both traditional Chinese and Western medical systems recognize that the kidneys play an essential role in filtering and expelling waste water. But Chinese medical theory discusses the organs based not only on their function but on their relationship with other organs. In traditional organ theory, the kidneys are also responsible for reproduction and fertility; this theory has no counterpart in the Western anatomic concept of the organ. Yet, herbs that nourish "kidney essence" are quite effective clinically in promoting fertility.

It is important to let each medical system stand on its own rather than attempting to create a one-to-one correspondence between Western anatomy and the Taoist functional organ systems. Each system has its own strengths and weaknesses, and each is complete in its own way.

THE YIN ORGANS

In traditional Chinese medicine, the five yin organs, or solid (zang) organs, are the lungs, spleen, heart, liver, and kidneys. The pericardium is sometimes considered a sixth yin organ. The yin organs produce, transform, and store qi, blood, body fluids, and essence.

THE LUNGS (FEI)

The lungs are considered the "tender organ" because they open directly to the external environment and are usually the first internal organ attacked by external pathogens such as bacteria. Symptoms of imbalance in the lungs include cough, asthma, phlegm, chest pain, bloating, loss of voice, and nosebleeds.

The functions of the lungs in traditional Chinese medicine:

The lungs control breathing. This important function closely parallels the Western understanding of the organ. In addition to controlling inhalation of oxygen and exhalation of carbon dioxide, the lungs—along with the spleen—are seen as the source of postnatal qi, the actual vitality of a person. (The kidneys are considered the source of prenatal qi, the constitution.) The concept of postnatal qi is important because people with a weak constitution don't have to be consigned to a lifetime of fatigue or illness. Through breathing exercises such as qi gong, a person can enhance vitality through the qi of the lungs.

The lungs control the qi of the entire body. Since the lungs transform inhaled air into qi, they have an important influence on the functional activities of the body. When lung qi is strong, breathing is normal and the body has sufficient energy. Weak lung qi, on the other hand, deprives the other organs and body tissues of energy, leading to shortness of breath, weak voice, and fatigue.

The lungs control body fluids in the lower part of the body. An organ of the upper body, the lungs assist in moving qi and body fluids to the lower portion of the body. When this descending action of the lungs is impaired and normal qi flow is disrupted, cough and shortness of breath may occur. Also, fluids can collect in the upper body, resulting in edema (severe water retention) and difficulty in urination. If this concept is difficult to understand from a Western anatomic perspective, think of it from an energetic perspective. For example, when you dip a drinking straw into water, the straw fills with water. The water then flows out of the straw when you lift the straw out of the water. However, if you place a finger over the end of the straw before you lift it out of the water, the water remains in the straw until you lift your finger. This action is similar to the blockage of downward water movement that results from impairment in lung function.

The lungs govern body hair and skin. This principle refers to the lungs' function of dispersing moisture to the skin, maintaining its suppleness and elasticity. The body hair and pores are also considered an integral part of the lungs' defensive system: They act as the boundary between the environment and the interior of the body. The qi that flows just under the skin is called wei qi and is considered the body's immune system. When the wei qi is strong, the body is able to fight off external pathogens. Clinically, the relationship between the lungs and the pores is seen in persons who frequently catch colds: They often complain that they have an aversion to wind, and they break into a sweat when they aren't feeling warm. These symptoms are due to an impairment of the lungs' control of the pores, resulting in the access to the body's interior by external pathogens.

The lungs open to the nose and control the voice. When lung qi is healthy, the sense of smell is acute, the nasal passages remain open, and the voice is strong. When lung qi experiences dysfunction, the person may experience symptoms of nasal congestion, excessive mucus, an impaired sense of smell, and a weak or hoarse voice. As most of us have experienced, a breakdown in energy throughout the body often follows these symptoms.

THE SPLEEN (PI)

Of all the organs in traditional Chinese medicine, the spleen bears the least resemblance to its Western counterpart. The latter deals primarily with production and destruction of red blood cells and storage of blood. In traditional Chinese physiology, the spleen plays a central part in the health and vitality of the body, taking a lead role in the assimilation of nutrients and maintenance of physical strength. It turns food from the stomach into nutrients and qi. Entire schools of medicine were formed around this organ; the premise was that all aspects of vitality depend on the entire body receiving proper nutrition from the healthy functioning of this essential organ. Symptoms of imbalance in the spleen include a lack of appetite, muscular atrophy (wasting), indigestion, abdominal fullness, bloating, jaundice, and inappropriate bleeding or bruising.

The traditional attributes possessed by the spleen:

The spleen governs transformation and transportation. Once the stomach breaks down and digests food, the spleen transforms it into usable nutrition and qi, then transports this food essence to the other organs. The spleen plays an essential role in the production of blood as well. For this reason, fatigue (qi deficiency) and anemia (blood deficiency) are often attributed to a breakdown in the spleen's ability to transform food into qi and blood. In addition to its role in nutrition and blood production, the spleen is also responsible for the "transformation of fluids": It assists in water metabolism, helping the body rid itself of excess fluid and moistening the areas that need it, such as the joints. If this function is disrupted, fluid disorders such as edema (severe water retention) or excessive phlegm can develop.

The spleen governs the blood. Considered the "foundation of postnatal existence," the spleen is the most important organ involved in production of sufficient blood to maintain health. A nutritious diet appropriate to the individual's needs enhances the qi of the spleen, thus improving the person's energy. These improvements are seen in clinical practice, where a sickly person can become quite strong through tonifying herbs, dietary changes, and breathing exercises. Spleen qi is also responsible for keeping blood within the vessels. A weakness in this function can lead to chronic bleeding, such as a tendency to bruise easily, or breakthrough bleeding in the middle of menstrual cycles.

The spleen dominates the muscles and four limbs. Since the spleen is responsible for transforming food into qi and blood and transporting them throughout the body, proper organ function is essential to maintain muscle mass and strong limbs. A person with deficient spleen qi often experiences weakness and fatigue in the limbs. Exercise and a healthy diet benefit the body only if the spleen is able to transmit nutrition and energy to the muscles.

The spleen opens into the mouth and lips. As the gateway to the digestive system, the mouth can indicate whether the spleen is functioning normally. If qi is normal, appetite is good, the lips are red and supple, and the sense of taste is sufficiently sensitive.

Spleen qi moves in an upward direction. All organs have a normal direction for their flow of qi. The flow of spleen qi keeps other organs in their proper place. If spleen qi is weak, then prolapse, or sagging, of the transverse colon, uterus, rectum, or stomach can result.

The spleen likes warmth and dislikes cold. Since the digestive enzymes require warmth to break down food properly, excessive consumption of cold foods and drinks can impair spleen function. Foods that are warming and easy to digest, such as soups with grated ginger, benefit spleen function.

THE HEART (XIN)

Known in traditional Chinese physiology as the ruler of the other organs, the heart has exceptional importance. Its function in traditional Chinese medicine parallels its Western anatomic function of pumping blood throughout the body to maintain life, but it is also intimately involved with mental and emotional processes. Considered the residence of the mind and spirit, the heart is the organ most often involved in psychological imbalances. Properly nourished and balanced, the heart maintains our innate wisdom, contentment, and emotional balance. Symptoms of heart imbalance include palpitations, shortness of breath, sweating easily, mental restlessness, insomnia, forgetfulness, chest pain, tongue pain, and burning urine.

The traditional functions of the heart:

The heart controls the blood and blood vessels. When the heart is healthy, it pumps blood vigorously through the vessels to all parts of the body, nourishing the organs and maintaining vitality. A deficiency in this function can appear as pale complexion, cold hands and feet, palpitations, insomnia, and emotional disturbances.

The heart manifests on the face. When the heart is strong and possesses sufficient blood, the complexion is rosy, and the individual looks robust and healthy. When the heart blood is deficient, on the other hand, the person looks pale and unhealthy. If heart yang or qi is deficient, the complexion may appear bluish, especially in the lips.

The heart houses the shen (spirit) and mind. This function encompasses the full range of human consciousness, including emotional health, mental function, memory, and spirituality. When the yin of the heart is deficient, a person can experience symptoms such as palpitations, anxiety, insomnia, and restlessness. When the heart blood is deficient, poor memory, depression, and a tendency to be "spaced out" or "in the clouds" can result.

The heart opens onto the tongue. In Chinese physiology, when an internal organ opens onto a sensory organ, it means the two organs are linked through structure, function, or physiology. By examining the sensory organ, a practitioner can determine much about the health of the internal organ linked to it. The tongue can indicate health or imbalance in all the organs. A pale tongue can indicate heart blood deficiency, while a red tongue with no coating may indicate heart yin deficiency. On another level, "the heart controls speech." Heart deficiency syndromes can lead to a withdrawn demeanor, for example. One patient who sought acupuncture treatment had experienced a complete loss of voice after a traumatic experience. While receiving stimulation in a heart channel point on the wrist, the patient got angry and shouted, "Do you realize how much that hurts?" After apologizing to the patient, the practitioner reminded him that he had just spoken for the first time in a week! This sort of dramatic release of emotional trauma is quite common in acupuncture therapy.

THE LIVER

The liver plays an important role. Since it is in charge of the smooth flow of qi throughout the body, any disruption in its functions usually affects another organ. Stagnation of the flow of liver qi frequently disrupts emotional flow, producing feelings of frustration or anger. Conversely, these same emotions can lead to a dysfunction in the liver, resulting in a loop of cause and effect.

Associated with the storage of blood, the liver is also the primary organ involved in a woman's menstrual cycle. When the liver is out of balance, the following symptoms can occur: emotional problems, rib pain or fullness, dizziness, headache, cramping, tendon problems, menstrual problems, jaundice, weak or blurry vision, and digestive disorders.

The functions of the liver:

The liver stores the blood. The liver is considered a storage area for blood when blood is not being used for physical activity. These periods of rest contribute to the body's restorative processes. During exercise, the blood is released to nourish the tendons and muscles. This function is also intimately associated with the menstrual cycle; the liver maintains an adequate blood supply and regulates the timing and comfort of menstruation. Any dysfunctions in the menstrual cycle are almost always treated through the regulation of liver blood, qi, or yin. When liver qi is stagnant (a very common condition), a person experiences irritability, tightness in the chest, and, in a woman, symptoms of premenstrual syndrome. When liver blood is deficient, symptoms such as dry eyes and skin, pallor, and lack of menstruation can occur.

The liver ensures the smooth flow of qi. The *Nei Jing* refers to the liver as a general in the army, coordinating troop movement. When the liver functions smoothly, so does physical and emotional activity throughout the body. When the liver's ability to spread qi smoothly throughout the body is disrupted due to stress or lifestyle choices, however, the liver qi can become either stagnant or hyperactive, causing havoc in other organs, such as the lungs, stomach, and spleen. Stress-related problems such as irritable bowel syndrome or indigestion can be successfully treated by working through the "smoothing of liver qi."

The liver controls the tendons. As discussed previously, the liver stores blood during periods of rest and then releases it to the muscles and tendons in times of activity. When liver blood is deficient, tightness and inflexibility in the muscles and tendons can result. If liver qi is stagnant, muscles can go into spasm. Such muscle spasms often occur when a person drinks strong coffee. Coffee, even the decaffeinated variety, is one of the most disruptive substances in relation to the smooth flow of liver qi.

The liver opens into the eyes. Although all the organs have some connection to the health of the eyes, the liver is connected to proper eye function. Chronic eye problems can usually be traced to a deficiency of liver yin or blood, for example. It is quite common to resolve eye disorders successfully by treating the liver.

The liver shows on the nails. When liver blood is plentiful, it spreads to the farthest areas of the body, including the fingernails and toenails. When liver blood is deficient, on the other hand, nails can appear pale, weak, and brittle.

THE KIDNEYS (SHEN)

Although the kidneys' function of regulating water metabolism in Chinese physiology closely parallels their function in Western medicine, their influence is much more far-reaching. They are the storage place for vital essence (jing), a subtle substance responsible for growth, development, reproduction, and fertility. They are also considered the source of yin and yang for all the other organs, so a chronic disruption in their function can potentially affect any other part of the body. The kidneys are the source of prenatal qi, which is inherited from the parents and interpreted as a person's innate constitution. Ultimately, the health and strength of the kidneys is the major determining factor in a person's long-term vitality and longevity. Symptoms of imbalance in the kidneys include low back pain, infertility, impotence or excessive sexual desire, urinary problems, tinnitus or deafness, edema, or asthma.

The traditional functions of the kidneys:

The kidneys store essence (jing). Jing is a subtle substance that underlies all organic life processes. While it includes reproductive fluids, its scope goes far beyond this. There are two main types of essence: prenatal and postnatal. Prenatal essence is derived from the genetic material of the parents as well as the vitality of their lifestyle, habits, and nutrition. It is essentially a person's inherited constitution. Postnatal essence, on the other hand, is within a person's control because it is derived from food and air. It is possible for a person who has a weak prenatal essence to lead a vital and healthy life through the maintenance of a strong postnatal essence. A healthy diet and lifestyle, along with exercise and breathing practices, such as qi gong, are the means to achieving strong postnatal essence. In fact, a person with a weak constitution and a healthy lifestyle is better off than a person with a strong constitution and an unhealthy lifestyle. The latter often goes for years without any illness and then suddenly succumbs to cancer or heart disease. The person with weaker prenatal essence, on the other hand, is unable to get away with an unhealthy lifestyle because he or she gets immediate feedback in the form of illness or fatigue.

The kidneys control water metabolism. The balance of yin and yang in the kidneys determines the efficiency of water metabolism in the body. When kidney yang or kidney qi are deficient, excessive urination or edema (swelling due to severe fluid retention) may occur.

The kidneys grasp the qi. While the lungs are the body's major organ of respiration, the kidneys provide the "grasping" force that is necessary for full inhalation. When kidney yang or kidney qi is deficient, therefore, a person may suffer a difficulty in inhalation, as is experienced by people with asthma.

The kidneys control the bones. According to Chinese physiology, the kidneys are responsible for the development of strong bones. When the kidneys are deficient, a person may have brittle bones, repeated injuries, and poor dental health. The kidneys produce marrow and are connected to the brain. Marrow has a much broader function in traditional Chinese medicine than it has in Western medicine. In Chinese physiology, marrow is derived from essence, and it is the source of the substance that makes up the brain. Deficiencies in essence or marrow can appear in cases of mental retardation.

The kidneys open into the ear. This function has great clinical significance: Hearing difficulties can often be treated by nourishing the kidneys. Babies are considered to have undeveloped hearing capacity due to the lack of maturation of kidney energy; elderly people tend to have ringing in the ears (tinnitus) or impaired hearing due to a depletion of their kidney qi over time.

THE PERICARDIUM (XIN BAO)

The pericardium provides a shield around the heart to protect it against external pathogenic factors. Sometimes considered a sixth yin organ, it has no separate functions of its own.

YANG ORGANS

The six yang organs, or hollow (fu) organs, are considered to be less significant in their functions than are the yin organs. The yang organs serve primarily to separate impure substances from food and then drain them out of the body. Each yang organ is paired with a yin organ. For example, the spleen and the stomach together encompass the digestive process. The stomach performs the yang function of processing the food and passing it on; the spleen performs the yin function of extracting nourishment from the food and transforming it into qi and blood.

THE STOMACH (WEI)

The stomach is the beginning of the digestive process, and its functions act as a yang complement to the spleen's yin functions. Symptoms of stomach dysfunction include excessive or impaired appetite, nausea, vomiting, excessive or insufficient thirst, and mouth sores.

The stomach is responsible for receiving and ripening food. The stomach functions as a cauldron in "rotting and ripening" food to prepare it for the spleen's extraction of its essence. Considered the "middle burner" when paired with the spleen, its proper functioning is essential for health and vitality.

The stomach controls digestion of food and water. If the stomach is weak in its ability to prepare food for digestion, the spleen is unable to create sufficient qi and blood, resulting in weakness or impairment in other organs.

Stomach qi moves downward. When the stomach qi functions properly, it has a downward movement. After the stomach separates the pure essence and transfers it to the spleen, the "rotted and ripened" (digested) food is sent downward to the small intestine for further processing. If this downward energy is disrupted, however, the stomach qi moves upward. Known as rebellious stomach qi, this upward movement produces symptoms of nausea, vomiting, belching, hiccups, and acid regurgitation (often called acid reflux in the West).

The stomach likes dampness and dislikes dryness. Since the stomach is a yang organ, it tends to overheat when it is out of balance. Maintaining a moist atmosphere with sufficient fluids in the stomach helps to ward off stomach yin deficiency. This can be achieved by avoiding alcohol, excessive spices, and dry foods that are consumed without fluids.

SMALL INTESTINE (XIAO CHANG)

The small intestine is paired with the heart in a yin/yang relationship. Symptoms of imbalance in the small intestine are lower abdominal pain, bloating, indigestion, gas, diarrhea, dark, burning urine, or blood in the urine.

The small intestine separates clear and dirty aspects of food and creates urine. After the stomach sends the pure essence of food to the spleen, it sends the rest to the small intestine. The spleen once again receives the "clear" aspect of the digested food, while the "dirty" part (the waste) is sent down to the large intestine. After food has been further processed, any impure fluids remaining are sent to the kidneys and bladder, where they are excreted as urine.

LARGE INTESTINE (DA CHANG)

The large intestine continues the process of digestion: It receives waste, absorbs fluids, and excretes feces. It is paired with the lungs. Disorders of the large intestine can lead to constipation, diarrhea, or lower abdominal pain.

The large intestine passes dirty qi and waste out of the body. After receiving the turbid material from the small intestine, the large intestine is the final stage of processing digested food. The final waste products of digestion are formed into stools and passed from the body.

The large intestine controls body fluids. As the final stage of fluid metabolism, the large intestine absorbs water from the products of digestion while forming stools. A disruption in this function can lead to diarrhea (too much fluid) or constipation (insufficient fluid).

URINARY BLADDER (PANG GUANG)

The urinary bladder's role is the same as it is in the West, storing urine and discharging it periodically. It is paired with the kidneys. Symptoms of bladder dysfunction include difficulty urinating, with burning, pain, urgency, bleeding, and retention.

The urinary bladder receives and excretes urine. After receiving turbid fluids from the lungs, small intestine, and large intestine, the kidneys extract the last of the pure essence. The remnants are then sent to the bladder, where they are stored until they are excreted from the body through urination.

GALLBLADDER (DAN)

The gallbladder is paired with the liver; liver disharmonies often affect the gallbladder and vice versa. Disharmonies of the gallbladder can produce symptoms such as intercostal pain (pain between the ribs), anger, rash decisions, timidity, digestive problems, and emotional disturbances.

The gallbladder stores and secretes bile. The liver produces bile and the gallbladder stores it. When you eat fatty foods, the gallbladder contracts and pours bile into the small intestine to assist in digestion. Overconsumption of fatty foods can adversely affect the function of the liver and gallbladder.

The gallbladder rules decisions. A timid person is said to have a weak gallbladder. A person who acts impulsively or out of anger, on the other hand, could be suffering from an excess yang condition in the gallbladder.

TRIPLE BURNER (SAN JIAO)

The triple burner is not an organ per se, but rather it is a grouping of organs by function and location. The triple burner is paired with the pericardium in a yin/yang relationship.

Upper Burner: Comprising the heart and lungs, the upper burner is described as a "fog" or "mist." It disperses the essence of food and qi throughout the body. Illness usually attacks this burner first, then proceeds to the middle and lower burners.

Middle Burner: The spleen and stomach function together as the middle burner, acting as a "foam." Metabolism in this burner involves churning food and water into a digestible, souplike consistency. Digestive disorders are often described as middle burner imbalances.

Lower Burner: The lower burner encompasses the organs below the navel: the intestines, kidneys, and bladder. It is considered a "swamp," since it is the sewage system of the body, excreting waste.

THE EXTRA OR "CURIOUS" ORGANS

The curious organs are so named because their existence can be confirmed through observation, but they don't fall into any category. They are the marrow, bones, blood vessels, brain, uterus, and gallbladder. Although the gallbladder is a yang organ, it is also considered a curious organ since it is the only yang organ that stores a vital substance (bile). Marrow is a vital essence stored by the kidneys. It is related to growth and development and nourishes the brain. The functions of the other organs parallel their Western counterparts.

DISHARMONY

Over the centuries, a sophisticated system of diagnosis has evolved in traditional Chinese medicine. By following various established diagnostic procedures, a practitioner of traditional Chinese medicine can construct a detailed picture of the status of all the internal organs without the aid of laboratory tests or other types of modern technology. To identify a pattern of disharmony, the physician will assess the status of the organs, gradually uncovering the cause of the disease by grouping the symptoms into traditional patterns.

TRADITIONAL PATTERNS OF DISHARMONY

During the initial patient visit, the practitioner must organize all of the seemingly unrelated facts gathered about a patient's condition, gradually refining this information into diagnostic categories. At first, the practitioner organizes the evidence loosely into general categories known as the eight parameters, which consist of four groups of polarities: yin and yang, heat and cold, internal and external, excess and deficiency. This eight-parameter diagnosis is the basic foundation for all diagnostic categories. It gives the practitioner a general overview of the patient's disease, or pattern of disharmony. Once the practitioner has grouped the symptoms according to the eight parameters, he or she can further refine the diagnosis to determine the condition of the vital substances and internal organs. In this way, the diagnosis evolves from a general image into a specific, clear description of the individual patient's physiologic processes. For example, in organ diagnosis, spleen qi deficiency is a pattern of disharmony. This is a very specific diagnosis. In eight-parameter diagnosis, the same imbalance is classified generally as a deficient internal condition.

THE EIGHT PARAMETERS

It's important to remember that in traditional Chinese medicine, illness is seen as an imbalance, a lack of harmony in the body's systems. This disharmony is understood in terms of the eight principal parameters. Knowledge of the eight parameters allows the practitioner to perceive the location, severity, and nature of the disease process. This information is then applied to the other diagnostic categories of qi, blood, and internal organs, further narrowing and focusing the diagnosis. It is also important to remember that a physical condition is not fixed; inner processes are always subject to change. In other words, a yin condition can evolve into a yang condition; an exterior pattern can penetrate to the interior; a cold condition might turn to heat; and an excess disease often becomes one of deficiency. In a more complex disharmony, all eight patterns could occur simultaneously! For this reason, it is always a good idea to maintain a Taoist attitude of flexibility while perceiving the movements of nature. Any diagnostic pattern is simply a snapshot in time; an experienced practitioner recognizes this and is always prepared to adjust the diagnosis and treatment plan to accommodate these changes.

EXTERNAL/INTERNAL

The terms external (or exterior) and internal (or interior) do not refer to where the pathogen comes from; rather, they specify the location of the disease process in the body. The exterior of the body is considered the skin and muscles, while the interior is defined as the internal organs and bones. In an external pattern, the pathogen fights with the body's defensive qi, or wei qi, which circulates under the skin. Symptoms of this struggle are chills, fever, sensitivity to wind or cold, body aches, sore throat, nasal congestion, and a floating pulse. If the cause of disease, known in traditional Chinese medicine as the pernicious influence, is not expelled, typically it penetrates the interior. An interior, or internal, condition has more organ-related symptoms, such as diarrhea, stomachache, intestinal cramps, lung pain, bladder pain, constipation, and changes in the color of the tongue. A pathogen trapped between the interior and exterior exhibits such symptoms as alternating chills and fever, a bitter taste in the mouth, and a wiry pulse.

HEAT/COLD

The possible causes of heat conditions are an external heat pernicious influence (for example, a virus that produces heat symptoms, such as a high fever), internal hyperactivity of yang functions (for example, drinking too much alcohol can cause a red face and headache), or insufficient yin. The yin aspect of the body includes the "lubricating and cooling" systems. When these systems are depleted, the body tends to overheat due to the deficiency of yin. In general, heat signs include redness in the face; feeling hot; thirst; colored secretions (such as yellow mucus or other discharges or dark urine); constipation; burning sensations; irritability; red tongue body with a yellow coating; and a rapid pulse.

Conversely, cold arises from external cold pernicious influences (for example, a virus that produces the cold symptoms of chills and a runny nose), an internal yang deficiency, or internal excess cold pathogenic factors. An internal yang deficiency produces such symptoms as always feeling cold, a low sex drive, and low energy. A person who has acute symptoms of loose stools and abdominal pains from eating too much ice cream likely has an internal excess cold condition. General signs of cold are a pale face, feelings of cold, lack of thirst, clear secretions (pale urine, clear mucus or discharges), loose stools, muscle tightness, fatigue, pale tongue with a white coating, and a slow pulse.

EXCESS/DEFICIENCY

A disease is classified as an excess condition or a deficient condition. Excess conditions occur when an external pernicious influence attacks the body and creates overactivity (for example, a high fever that is caused by infection with a virus); a body function becomes overactive (for example, redness and swelling that are caused by an infection); or an obstruction of qi or blood causes pain. Acute conditions tend to be conditions of excess. Deficient conditions arise due to an inherent weakness in the body or a weakness in the body's vital energy (qi), blood, yin, or yang. Symptoms of deficiency include weak movement, pale face, pale tongue, and weak pulse. Chronic conditions tend to be conditions of deficiency.

YIN/YANG

The most general of all the diagnostic categories, it can be considered a summary of all the others. Heat, excess, and external conditions are yang conditions, while cold, deficiency, and internal conditions are yin conditions. Most conditions include a mixture of yin and yang imbalances. In addition, each internal organ has its yin and yang aspects that must be balanced. For example, if heart yin is deficient, a person may experience insomnia, poor memory, and palpitations. If heart yang is depleted, poor circulation, pale face, purple lips, edema, and cold extremities can result. When yin, with its cooling function, is low, heat signs occur. When yang, with its heating function, is low, cold signs occur. Restoring the optimum yin/yang balance of each internal organ is the most important secret of maintaining health in traditional Chinese medicine.

SYNDROMES OF QI, BLOOD, YIN, AND YANG

Analyzing disease according to the eight parameters is essential in arriving at a diagnosis. However, it is only the first step; it usually does not provide enough information for a focused treatment. A person might have chronic fatigue—according to the eight parameters, chronic fatigue indicates an internal deficiency. The practitioner might recognize at this point that the person needs tonifying herbs to nourish and alleviate the deficiency, but which herbs? With further inquiry, the practitioner learns that the person also has loose stools and a poor appetite. Since these symptoms are related to the functions of spleen qi, the practitioner now knows that the syndrome is an internal deficiency of spleen qi. By combining the eight parameters with knowledge of the vital substances and the organs, the diagnosis is now detailed enough to make a focused treatment plan. Tonifying herbs improve overall function of a particular organ and strengthen the entire organism when used long term.

Remember that qi flows in a system of channels, called meridians, in the body, and each organ is linked to a meridian. Acupuncture can affect or manipulate qi to treat a specific imbalance. A practitioner might choose herbs that tonify spleen qi and use acupuncture or moxibustion (the application of heat) at acupuncture points that affect the spleen. For example, a point on the spleen meridian known as Spleen 6 can be activated to strengthen the spleen. Since the spleen and stomach meridians are directly connected, needling or applying moxibustion to a point on the stomach meridian (Stomach 36) also strengthens the spleen. In this way, a wide variety of treatment options are available to a practitioner once an accurate diagnosis is at hand.

DISORDERS OF QI

There are four disorders of qi: deficient qi, stagnant qi, sinking qi, and rebellious qi. When qi is deficient, the principal symptoms are fatigue, a bright pale face, a weak or soft voice, spontaneous sweating, a pale tongue, and a weak pulse. These general symptoms could occur in any type of qi deficiency. The treatment is to tonify qi.

Another type of qi imbalance is stagnant qi, an excess type of disharmony. Since health depends on the smooth flow of qi, stagnant qi can cause discomfort or pain almost anywhere in the body. It is typically associated with feelings of pain or distention that move from place to place, irritability, and soft lumps anywhere on the body that come and go. Premenstrual syndrome is a condition of stagnant qi in the liver. The treatment principle is to smooth the flow of qi through the affected organs or meridians.

In the disorder of sinking qi, a deficiency syndrome, the function of supporting the organs is impaired. Prolapse (sagging) of the bladder, rectum, transverse colon, or uterus occurs. Herbs that have an uplifting action, along with acupuncture and moxibustion, are used to treat this condition.

Finally, in patterns of rebellious qi, the flow of qi is the reverse of normal. For example, the normal direction of flow for stomach qi is downward. When rebellious stomach qi occurs, symptoms of nausea, vomiting, belching, or hiccups exist. The treatment principle is to return the flow of qi to normal, usually with herbs and acupuncture treatments. It is also necessary to rectify any underlying excess or deficiency that caused the problem.

DISORDERS OF BLOOD

Three types of blood disorders can occur: deficiency, stagnation, and excess of heat. Blood deficiency syndrome is especially common among women due to their monthly loss of menstrual blood. It can also arise as a result of improper nutrition or spleen qi deficiency, which prevents full assimilation of nutrients. Symptoms include a dull pale face, pale lips, pale tongue, dizziness, blurry vision, numbness or tingling of extremities, poor memory, dry skin and hair, scanty menses, and a thin pulse. The treatment principle is to tonify the blood with herbs, acupuncture, or moxibustion.

In blood stagnation, which is an excess pattern, the primary symptom is a fixed, stabbing pain, which can occur anywhere in the body as a result of injury, stagnation of qi or cold, or deficient blood conditions. Tumors or painful menstrual flow with clots may also occur. The treatment depends on the nature of the stagnation, but the common treatment principle is to activate or move the blood with herbs that stimulate circulation. Acupuncture is especially effective in treating the pain resulting from the stagnation.

With an excess condition of heat in the blood, symptoms of hemorrhage, skin rashes, itchiness, blood mixed in with bodily secretions, irritability, and sensations of heat can occur. Treatment includes using herbs that cool the blood along with hemostatic herbs to stop the bleeding.

DISORDERS OF YIN

In disorders of yin deficiency, the cooling, moistening action of the body is depleted, leading to symptoms of reddish cheeks, red tongue with little or no coat, dry throat, heat in the "five palms" (palms, soles, and sternum; sometimes called "five hearts"), night sweats, irritability, and a small, rapid pulse. The presence of additional symptoms depends on the organ system affected. The treatment principle is to tonify the yin and clear deficiency heat. In conditions of yin excess, there can be feelings of cold, mucus, and a general sluggishness. Treatment varies, depending on the particular type of excess yin, but it usually involves the use of warming herbs or diuretics.

DISORDERS OF YANG

Yang deficiency is a chronic syndrome characterized by cold extremities, lack of sexual desire, infertility, an aversion to cold, pale face, tongue, and lips, and a slow, weak pulse. Other signs and symptoms depend on the particular organ systems affected. The treatment principle is to tonify the yang. In yang excess disorders, signs and symptoms include headache, body aches, fever, sweating, thirst, red eyes, concentrated urine, constipation, mental restlessness, a red tongue with a yellow coating, and a full, rapid pulse. In this condition, the treatment principle is to clear excess heat.

THE CAUSES OF DISHARMONY

Practitioners of traditional Chinese medicine consider a number of factors in determining the cause of illness. Some of these causes are considered external, as in the six pernicious influences: wind, cold, heat, dryness, dampness, and summer heat. Other causes are considered internal, as in the seven emotions: anger, joy, worry, pensiveness, sadness, fear, and shock. Other factors that play a role in the development of disease are diet, lifestyle, and accidents. When the body is healthy, its various substances and energies are in harmonious balance, both internally and in relation to the external environment. When this innate vitality (true qi) and immune defenses (wei qi) are strong, it is difficult for externally contracted disease to gain a foothold, especially if the invading pathogen is weak. However, an exceptionally strong pathogen can overwhelm a healthy person, especially if the person has been weakened by stress, fatigue, overwork, or other lifestyle factors. For example, a person with a strong immune system might avoid catching a cold, even if a sick person sneezes on him. However, if he drinks a test tube full of the same virus, his strong immune system will be no match for such an onslaught. On the other hand, a person with very weak wei qi can catch whatever pathogen may be around due to his or her exceptionally weak defenses. This is the reason the elderly and young children are most at risk during influenza epidemics.

THE SIX PERNICIOUS INFLUENCES

Also known as the six pathogenic factors, six excesses, or six evils, these are the causes of disease that often arise from outside the body. They are wind, cold, heat, dampness, dryness, and summer heat. Although Western medicine recognizes only viruses and bacteria as external pathogens, the Chinese observed that the body mirrors certain climatic conditions. (This follows the Taoist principle that "the macrocosm is within the microcosm.") Although a diagnosis of "wind and cold invading the lungs" might sound primitive, this type of diagnosis accurately describes the way a certain type of pathogenic factor behaves inside the human body. The wind symptoms act just like wind in nature: They come and go, often without warning. Similarly, the cold symptoms act as they do in nature: They cause contraction, they slow functions down, and they make the person feel cold.

The high degree of effectiveness in treating this type of disorder (such as with herbs that "repel wind and scatter cold") is proof that the diagnosis is much more than a mere philosophical idea. Although Western medicine might be able to isolate the virus causing this condition, it still has no safe and effective way of treating the virus, other than relieving some of the symptoms it causes. On the other hand, thousands of years of trial and error through observation of nature and the human body have led to numerous effective treatments in Chinese medicine for viral infections that fit this pattern.

When learning about and discussing the various internal "climates" of the human body, it is important to remember that they may not always match the external climate. It is quite common for a person to develop symptoms of cold and dampness in rainy winter weather, but it is also possible to develop heat symptoms under the same weather conditions. Illness is the combination of the particular pathogen involved and a person's unique response to it. It is also possible for the pernicious influences to arise from internal causes. In this case, they usually result from a chronic internal imbalance. Descriptions of the six pernicious influences follow.

WIND

The pernicious influence of wind is considered the major cause of illness in traditional Chinese patterns of disharmony. It combines readily with other pathogens, giving rise to syndromes known as wind cold, wind heat, and wind dampness. This pathogenic factor possesses the qualities of wind in nature, appearing without warning and constantly changing. Considered a yang form of evil qi, it often attacks the upper body, head, throat, and eyes. Wind causes movement, so it is usually involved when there are symptoms of twitching, spasms, or shaking. The organ most often affected by external wind is the lung; internal wind most commonly is related to an imbalance in the liver.

SYNDROMES OF WIND

Wind Cold: In this syndrome, the pernicious influence of wind combines with that of cold. The person experiences symptoms of chills, fever (which is less severe than the chills), no sweating, headache, nasal congestion, and stiffness and pain in the shoulders, upper back, neck, and occipital area (back of the head). Cold causes objects to contract, and its effects in the body are no different. It causes chills, and the shivering causes the muscles to become tight and stiff. Although actual shivering may not occur, the person has difficulty staying warm, even when dressed properly for the conditions. Wind cold is traditionally treated with warm, diaphoretic (sweat-inducing) herbs to disperse the cold and repel the wind.

Wind Heat: Caused by a combination of pathogens, this syndrome is seen typically in the common cold or flu. The person may have symptoms of red face, high fever, sore throat, red eyes, thirst, red tongue, and a rapid pulse. Treatment for wind heat syndrome includes herbs that clear heat and repel wind.

Wind Damp: Arthritis is a manifestation of this pattern. Like dampness in nature, which is persistent and requires time to eradicate, the dampness pathogenic influence is difficult to cure and takes some time to resolve. The influence of wind also causes the pain to migrate from joint to joint, sometimes disappearing for a while only to reappear without warning. Treatment for this syndrome includes herbs that drain dampness and improve circulation of qi and blood through the affected areas. Moxibustion therapy—the application of heat—is particularly helpful in this situation.

Wind Water: This is a sudden attack of edema (swelling due to severe fluid retention), usually from allergies, poisoning, or acute nephritis (inflammation of the kidney). Diaphoretic (sweat-inducing) or diuretic (urine-producing) herbs are used along with acupuncture and moxibustion to treat this condition. The herbs help the body eliminate fluid, moxibustion helps the body metabolize fluids and improves circulation, and acupuncture moves stagnant fluids and expels the pathogenic factor.

Wind Rash: This category includes any skin condition that appears suddenly. Since dampness often plays a role in this condition, it can be difficult to treat. Treatment can include herbs that "scatter wind, clear heat, and drain dampness." For example, if the rash is red and burns, herbs that clear heat are also used. Monitoring the diet is always an essential part of treatment. Coffee, in particular, should be avoided in skin conditions, since it heats up the blood, further increasing the wind.

Liver Wind Moving Internally: This is an internal condition of the liver that can result from a long-term imbalance; the usual chronic patterns are liver yin deficiency or blood deficiency. Signs of this condition are various abnormal body movements, such as twitching, shaking, convulsions, and spasms. The liver is in charge of the smooth movement of qi and blood in the body as well as harmonious movement within the body. An imbalance in the liver impairs this function, producing abnormal movement, and the influence of wind stirs this movement at unpredictable times.

Excessive Heat Producing Wind: If heat is too extreme, it can cause a sudden collapse, as in heatstroke. It can also cause sudden convulsions, such as those that occur in children with a high fever. Compare this internal process with what happens in nature when rising hot air causes gusts of high wind.

Blood Deficiency Leading to Wind: Since the liver stores blood, a deficiency of blood affects the liver, leading to wind. This can produce numbness and cramping. When the blood is tonified, these symptoms disappear.

COLD

The cold pathogenic factor is considered a yin evil qi. Its nature is to slow movement down, causing tightness, contraction, stagnation, and impaired circulation. When it is an external pathogenic factor, cold can attack the skin, muscles, and lungs. When it is an internal pathogenic factor, cold can cause an impairment in the normal functions of the spleen, stomach, and kidneys.

SYNDROMES OF COLD

Wind Cold: In combination with the pathogenic factor of wind, cold attacks the exterior of the body and the lungs, causing chills, lack of sweating, occipital headache (pain at the base of the skull), upper body aches, tight shoulders and neck, and a congested nose. The influence of wind causes the symptoms to appear suddenly and affect the upper body, while cold causes the muscles to contract, causing the stiffness and pain. Nasal secretions are clear—another sign of cold. The treatment principle is to repel the wind and disperse the cold with warm diaphoretic herbs, acupuncture, and moxibustion.

Obstruction Due to Cold: Traditionally known as cold bi pain, this condition typically takes the form of body aches or joint pain that is relieved by warmth. The most common Western diagnosis for this is arthritis. Since the syndrome is caused by cold, the joint may actually feel cold to the touch, and the pain typically gets worse in cold weather. The Chinese treatment principle is to increase circulation and warm the acupuncture meridians through which qi and blood circulate by means of moxibustion, acupuncture, and herbs.

Cold Attacking the Spleen and Stomach: In this externally caused disorder, cold causes digestive symptoms such as abdominal pain, clear vomit, and watery diarrhea. Although it usually accompanies an externally contracted cold or stomach bacteria or virus (what we commonly refer to as stomach "flu"), this syndrome can also be caused by eating cold foods such as ice cream.

Cold Congealing the Liver Meridian: The liver meridian passes through the genital area, and this condition is a manifestation of cold in that meridian. Symptoms include testicular pain or shrinking and hernia pain. Moxibustion, acupuncture, and herbs can effectively correct this imbalance in a short time.

Spleen Yang Deficiency: If a person has an underlying deficiency of spleen yang (deficiency in energy and heat needed in order to digest food), cold can severely impair digestive function. Symptoms of spleen yang deficiency include watery stools with undigested food, cold extremities, edema, and a slow pulse. When a person with this underlying deficiency is also affected by external cold pathogens, the imbalance is especially difficult to eliminate. Treatment first expels the cold pathogenic factor. Then it tonifies the yang aspect of the spleen and kidneys to bring about a long-term increase in the body's basic metabolism, or its ability to maintain the heat needed for proper digestion, which is known in traditional Chinese medicine as life-gate (metabolic) fire. Spleen yang deficiency is treated with moxibustion and warming herbs that tonify spleen yang.

Kidney Yang Deficiency: Since the kidneys are the source of yang metabolic fire for the entire body, a deficiency in kidney yang can make the individual especially prone to cold. The symptoms of kidney yang deficiency include an inability to stay warm, cold extremities, low sex drive, frequent urination, edema (fluid retention), and pain in the low back. The yang deficiency can be corrected with long-term application of moxibustion and consumption of herbs that tonify kidney yang, thereby increasing metabolic fire.

HEAT

Heat, or fire, is a yang pernicious influence. As in nature, heat causes expansion and in-creased activity. When out of balance, heat can lead to irritability, fever, and inflammatory conditions. By its nature, heat rises, appearing as a red face and eyes, sore throat, and dizziness. If heat affects the heart or liver, anger may result. Heat tends to affect the body fluids, leading to thirst, constipation, and dark urine. Since it can produce wind, heat can lead to spasms.

SYNDROMES OF HEAT

Wind Heat: This very common condition appears mostly as the common cold and flu. Wind combines with heat to produce symptoms of fever, sore throat, thirst, headache, sweating, rapid pulse, and sometimes a red tip of the tongue. The treatment principle is to repel the wind and clear the heat with acupuncture and herbal formulas.

Excess Heat in the Organs: Symptoms of this yang excess condition are, typically, irritability, thirst, dry throat, concentrated (dark or burning) urine, constipation, red tongue with a yellow coat, and a full, rapid pulse. Other symptoms depend on the organ affected. For example, heart fire produces severe emotional disturbances; stomach fire can cause mouth ulcers; liver fire might stir up extreme anger; lung fire might bring about an accumulation of yellow mucus in the lungs. In all cases, the treatment is to clear the excess heat with herbs and with manipulation of acupuncture points that have an affinity for the organ affected.

Deficiency Heat: This syndrome is caused by a deficiency in the yin, cooling aspect of an organ; the resulting imbalance causes heat to flare up. The general symptoms of deficiency heat are red cheeks, night sweats, irritability, chronic inflammation, red tongue with no coat, and a thin, rapid pulse. Other symptoms depend on the organ affected. When the kidneys have deficiency heat, chronic urinary tract infections can occur; deficiency heat in the lungs—which can arise from cigarette smoking—can lead to a chronic dry cough; and the heat from heart yin deficiency can cause insomnia.

DAMPNESS

In nature, dampness soaks the ground and everything that comes in contact with it, and stagnation results. Once something becomes damp, it can take a long time for it to dry out again. The yin pathogenic influence of dampness has similar qualities: It is persistent and heavy, and it can be difficult to resolve. A person who spends a lot of time in the rain, lives in a damp environment, or sleeps on the ground may be susceptible to external dampness. Similarly, a person who eats large amounts of ice cream, cold foods and drinks, greasy foods, and sweets is prone to imbalances of internal dampness.

Dampness has tangible and intangible aspects. Tangible dampness includes phlegm, edema, and discharges. Intangible dampness includes subjective feelings of heaviness and dizziness. A "slippery" pulse and a greasy tongue usually accompany both types of dampness. In general, symptoms of dampness in the

AN ORGAN IN DISHARMONY

Each organ has a preferred internal environment, which supports its optimum functional abilities. The spleen is especially vulnerable to the influence of cold and dampness, for example, both in the external climate and in the diet. Since the spleen is the most important organ involved in digestion, this preference can be seen when a person eats too much cold, raw food. For example, ice cream is cold and it promotes dampness since it is both sweet and a dairy product. A person who eats too much ice cream, especially in cold weather, often has poor digestion and loose stools. When the spleen is cold and damp, it also causes the body to produce excessive mucus, which then overwhelms the lungs, leading to frequent colds, asthma, and allergies. (If you have ever coughed up mucus after eating ice cream, you have experienced the way cold produces dampness.)

On the other hand, hot, cooked foods nourish the spleen, especially when combined with warming, drying herbs such as ginger or black pepper. Eating foods such as this, especially in cold weather, leads to strong digestion, and the body produces less mucus, making the person less susceptible to colds and other respiratory ailments. If an organ's optimum functional environment is maintained, the organ will perform efficiently, contributing to the health of the entire body.

body include water retention, swelling, feelings of heaviness, coughing phlegm, and skin rashes that ooze or are crusty. Since dampness is heavy, it has a tendency to sink downward to affect the lower parts of the body: A person may experience a feeling of sinking or heaviness, and swelling frequently affects the legs. These characteristics are the opposite of wind, which has a tendency to affect the upper part of the body. When dampness combines with heat, the condition of damp heat develops, which can cause such symptoms as burning urine, sticky foul-smelling stools, yellow vaginal discharges, and jaundice.

SYNDROMES OF DAMPNESS

Wind Damp: This form of the common cold is characterized by chills, headache, afternoon fever, nausea, and diarrhea. A person may describe feeling as if a wet towel is wrapped around the head. Treatment includes moxibustion and herbs that repel wind.

Wind Damp Joint Pain: This condition is characterized by a dull and heavy pain and numbness that can persist in certain joints. Rheumatic pain that gets worse in damp weather is a good example of this type of imbalance. The condition tends to be chronic and resistant to treatment. Treatment with acupuncture and moxibustion can relieve the stiffness and pain. Herbs that clear wind damp, such as mulberry branches (sang zhi) and cinnamon twigs (gui zhi), are used to decrease swelling and improve circulation, following the Chinese principle of using "branches (tree limbs) to treat branches (body limbs)."

Damp and Toxins on the Skin: This condition includes any skin inflammation that also has a weepy, damp nature, such as eczema, skin ulcers, and allergic reactions that produce a discharge (skin eruptions that ooze or that are crusty). Herbs are used both internally and in the form of topical poultices.

Internal Dampness: Typically due to an imbalance in the spleen, symptoms of internal dampness include bloating, diarrhea, lack of appetite, undigested food in the stools, fatigue, and possible edema in the abdominal area. When a person coughs up mucus right after eating ice cream, it shows that a cold spleen produces dampness. Since excessive dampness in the spleen is stored in the lungs, a damp spleen can often lead to frequent colds and allergies. Treatment of internal dampness focuses on eliminating the dampness with diuretic herbs and activating the spleen with tonifying herbs.

DRYNESS

Dryness is a yang pernicious influence. It is associated with the autumn season due to the lack of humidity in most areas at that time of year. Its influence on the body is drying and astringent.

It can easily deplete the body fluids, causing constipation, dry cough, concentrated urine, dryness in the throat and nose, thirst, and dry skin. Dryness typically enters the body through the nose and mouth, quickly affecting the lungs.

SUMMER HEAT

Summer heat is a yang pernicious influence that typically occurs in the heat and humidity of summer. It is "uprising and spread out," meaning it affects the head, causing thirst, red face, and headache, and it causes a person to lie down with the limbs spread out. The excessive sweating also leads to dark, concentrated urine, and depletion of the body's yin can occur. The extreme heat also affects the heart, leading to restlessness or even coma in severe cases such as heatstroke. When summer heat combines with dampness due to humidity and overconsumption of sugary drinks, such as soft drinks, the spleen is also affected. This leads to a loss of appetite, nausea, vomiting, diarrhea, and fatigue.

Treatment of summer heat is complex, depending on the organs and additional pathogenic factors involved. Usually, herbs are used that clear excess heat from within the body along with herbs that moisten the interior. Two common foods that are very effective in the treatment of this pattern are watermelon (xi gua) and mung beans (lu dou). There is also a point behind the knees (Weizhong, Bladder 40) associated with clearing heat; holding ice behind the knees helps the body cool down quickly. When digestive disturbances occur due to a combination of dampness and summer heat, cooling herbs are combined with herbs that clear turbid dampness, such as patchouli (huo xiang).

THE SEVEN EMOTIONS

The interaction of emotions with the physical body is an essential aspect of traditional Chinese medicine. The seven basic emotions related to organ function are anger, joy, worry, pensiveness, sadness, fear, and shock (fright). Each organ has a corresponding emotion; imbalance of this emotion can affect the organ's function. In discussing the emotional aspect of the disease process, it is important to remember that it is normal to experience the full range of emotions. It is only when a particular emotion is experienced over a prolonged period or with particular intensity that it becomes a source of imbalance. It is obviously important for a person with severe emotional problems to get professional help from a trained psychotherapist. But even in these cases, the therapy is more effective when the corresponding organ imbalance is rectified.

ANGER

Anger is associated with the liver. By its nature, anger causes qi to rise, leading to a red face and red eyes, headaches, and dizziness. This matches the pattern of liver fire rising. Anger can also cause liver qi to "attack the spleen," producing lack of appetite, indigestion, and diarrhea. In a more long-term view, suppressed anger or frustration often causes liver qi to become stagnant; this might result in depression or menstrual disorders. It is interesting to note that people who take herbs to release stagnant liver qi often experience bouts of anger as the stagnation is relieved. Similarly, anger and irritability are often the determining factor in diagnosing liver qi stagnation. Many people are relieved to know their rage has a physiologic basis. It is essential to avoid drinking coffee when treating anger-related liver disorders, as coffee heats the liver and greatly intensifies the condition.

JOY

A disorder related to joy may sound perplexing, since most people want as much joy as possible. The disorders from this emotion are not caused by happiness; rather, the imbalance comes from too much excitement or good news that comes as a shock to the system. When evaluating stress levels, psychologists look at all sources of stress, both positive and negative. Clearly the death of a spouse or a job loss is a significant source of stress. However, a marriage or job promotion, while a happy occasion, is also a source of stress. A person who is constantly on the go, living a life of excess can eventually develop heart imbalances with palpitations, anxiety, and insomnia. A person with heart imbalances may also exhibit emotional symptoms, since the heart is the seat of the spirit. A person with extreme disturbances of heart shen might be seen chattering happily to himself with outbursts of laughter. Such behavior results from the heart organ's inability to provide a stable resting place for the spirit. This imbalance is treated with acupuncture along the heart meridian. Herbal treatments consist of formulas that nourish heart blood or yin. If heart fire disturbs the spirit, herbs that clear heat from the heart are used.

WORRY

A very common emotion in our stress-filled society, worry can deplete the energy of the spleen. This can cause digestive disturbances and eventually lead to chronic fatigue: A weakened spleen cannot efficiently turn food into qi, and the lungs are unable to extract qi from air efficiently. A person who worries too much "carries the weight of the world on her shoulders," a good description of how a person feels when her weak spleen qi leads to dampness. Treatment would include moxa and herbs that strengthen the spleen, allowing a person the energy to deal with life's problems instead of dwelling on them.

PENSIVENESS

Too much thinking or obsessing about a topic can also deplete the spleen, causing a stagnation of its qi. A person with this condition may exhibit such symptoms as poor appetite, forgetting to eat, and bloating after eating. In time, the person may develop a pale complexion from a deficiency of spleen qi. This can eventually affect the heart, causing the person to dream about the same subjects at night. Students are often affected by this imbalance; the standard treatment is use of herbs that tonify heart blood and spleen qi.

SADNESS

Sadness or grief affects the lungs, producing fatigue, shortness of breath, crying, or depression. Treatment for this condition involves acupuncture to points along the lung and kidney meridians. Often, herbal formulas are used that tonify the qi or yin of the lungs.

FEAR

The emotion of fear is related to the kidneys. This relationship can readily be seen when extreme fear causes a person to urinate uncontrollably. In children, this can also manifest as bed-wetting, which psychologists have linked to insecurity and anxiety. Long-term anxiety due to worrying about the future can deplete the kidneys of yin, yang, and qi, eventually leading to chronic weakness. Treatment involves tonifying the kidneys with yin or yang tonics, depending on the particular symptoms.

SHOCK

Shock is especially debilitating to the kidneys and heart. The "fight or flight" reaction causes an excessive release of adrenaline from the adrenal glands that sit on top of the kidneys. This causes the heart to respond with palpitations, anxiety, and insomnia. Chronic stress from shock can be very debilitating to the entire system, causing a wide range of problems. Severe shock can have a long-term effect on the heart shen, as is evident in victims of post-traumatic stress syndrome. Treatment involves psychotherapy, herbs that calm the spirit and nourish the heart and kidneys, and regular acupuncture treatments.

DISORDERS OF THE INTERNAL ORGANS

It is important to remember that the functions of organs in traditional Chinese medicine may overlap those of their Western counterparts, but they also have totally unrelated functions. For this reason, it is dangerous to attempt to find a standard correspondence between the two. For example, a chest cold might be diagnosed as a lung condition under both systems, but asthma might be a kidney condition in traditional Chinese medical diagnostics. Both medical systems stand on their own strengths, but an attempt to artificially link the two can often make them less effective. Attempting to treat the flu simply with Chinese herbs that have antiviral qualities is less effective than getting an accurate diagnosis—wind heat, for example—and using a traditional formula for that wind heat.

The following section briefly describes the various conditions of imbalance that make up the foundation for an effective traditional treatment plan. Please keep in mind that many of these descriptions are for severe versions of the syndromes. The description of each pattern lists the full range of severity, from a mild set of symptoms to life-threatening disease. If intervention takes place at the early stages, it is possible to restore balance before the symptoms become more severe.

LUNG SYNDROMES

The lungs are in direct contact with the external environment; therefore, they are the organ most subject to attacks by external pernicious influences. They are also prone to disorders of yin deficiency and dryness, due to their need for a somewhat moist environment to function. (Each organ has its "favorite" climate, and a moist environment helps the lungs function.) Since the lungs govern qi, they affect the energy of the entire body if they become qi deficient.

Lung Qi Deficiency: This syndrome is characterized by shortness of breath, weak voice, spontaneous sweating, chronic weak cough, fatigue, bright pale face, frequent colds, a weak pulse, and a pale tongue. Some corresponding Western conditions might be asthma, emphysema, chronic bronchitis, allergies, depressed immune function, AIDS, and cancer. The treatment principle is to tonify lung qi with herbs such as ginseng (ren shen) and *Astragalus* (huang qi).

Lung Yin Deficiency: A chronic deficiency pattern, lung yin deficiency produces such symptoms as night sweats, fever, dry cough, small amounts of sticky phlegm or no phlegm, dry mouth, thirst, red cheeks, vocal distortions (weak voice, hoarseness, pitch changes), heat in the "five palms" (palms, soles, and sternum), red tongue with little or no coat, and a small rapid pulse. Western diagnoses are smoker's cough, tuberculosis, chronic sore throat, or chronic bronchitis. Treatment is to tonify lung yin and clear deficiency heat with herbs such as *Rehmannia* (sheng di huang) or *Ophiopogon* (mai men dong).

Wind Cold: This acute excess syndrome produces chills, possibly a mild fever, nasal congestion, headaches, upper body aches, a cough with clear or white phlegm that is easy to expectorate, and a tight, floating pulse. The common cold, acute bronchitis, and the early stages of pneumonia are considered to be wind cold conditions in traditional Chinese medicine. The treatment principle is to "release the exterior" with warm, diaphoretic herbs such as *Ephedra* (ma huang).

Wind Heat: This acute pattern differs somewhat from wind cold due to the influence of heat. Symptoms include a fever worse than the chills, a loud cough with yellow phlegm, sore throat, and a rapid, floating pulse. Treatment involves cooling herbs that release the exterior, such as honeysuckle (jin yin hua) or field mint (bo he).

Damp Phlegm Blocking the Lung: Copious amounts of clear or white phlegm is the main symptom of this excess syndrome. Other symptoms are shortness of breath, fullness in the chest, a thick, greasy tongue coating, slippery pulse, and a worsening of the symptoms when lying down. Corresponding Western conditions are chronic bronchitis with an acute episode, asthma, and bronchiectasis. Treatment involves herbs that clear phlegm from the lungs such as *Pinellia* (ban xia).

Hot Phlegm Stagnation: A serious internal excess pattern, hot phlegm stagnation produces such symptoms as difficulty breathing, thirst, a loud, frequent cough with green-yellow or bloody phlegm, a fishy smell on the breath, constipation, dark urine, chest pain, high fever, red tongue with a thick yellow coat, and a slippery, rapid pulse. Western diagnoses could be lung abscess, acute bronchitis, or pneumonia. Cooling antibiotic herbs, such as *Houttuynia* (yu xing cao) and *Scutellaria* (huang qin), are used.

Dryness Attacking the Lung: Symptoms of this syndrome include a dry cough, dry and cracked tongue coat, loss of voice, dry nose, sore, dry throat, and a floating, rapid pulse. Although it shares some aspects of yin deficiency, dryness attacking the lung is acute and external, while yin deficiency is chronic and internal. Another distinguishing factor is the lack of deficiency heat signs such as night sweats and "five palm heat." Some corresponding Western conditions are the common cold, acute bronchitis, later-stage pneumonia, allergy, and dehydration due to an overly dry environment. Herbs that moisten the lungs and release the exterior, such as *Phragmites* (lu gen) and kudzu (ge gen), are used.

SPLEEN SYNDROMES

The main functions of the spleen are to transform food and fluids, nourish the muscles, and control the blood, keeping it within the blood vessels. For this reason, most patterns of disharmony of the spleen involve poor appetite and digestion, fatigue, and bleeding disorders. The spleen prefers a dry environment, so it is prone to conditions of dampness from climate and dietary factors. It is especially sensitive to cold, damp weather and cold or raw foods, both of which are fertile ground for the pathogenic factor of dampness. When the spleen functions properly, the body is strong and well nourished. Blood, fluids, and the organs are also in their proper places; thus there is no deficient-type bleeding (blood), edema (fluids), or prolapse (organs).

Spleen Qi Deficiency: When the qi of the spleen is deficient, the spleen is unable to perform its functions of digestion. In addition to the typical qi deficiency signs of fatigue and pale face and tongue, additional symptoms specific to the spleen include poor appetite, weight loss, fullness and sleepiness after eating, and loose stools. (Other conditions are associated with spleen qi deficiency, such as sagging organs and bleeding, but these are discussed as separate syndromes.) Some corresponding Western conditions are ulcers, gastritis, chronic fatigue, AIDS, chronic indigestion, and hepatitis. Treatment consists of tonifying spleen qi with herbs such as ginseng (ren shen). The classic formula to tonify spleen qi is Four Gentlemen decoction (Si Jun Zi Tang).

Spleen Yang Deficiency: This more severe version of spleen qi deficiency has the above-mentioned symptoms as well as cold signs such as cold hands and feet, edema, a desire for warm food and drinks, abdominal discomfort after eating cold food, and diarrhea with undigested food in the stools. Western diseases that fit this syndrome are chronic gastroenteritis, infection with Candida, food allergies, and chronic hepatitis. The treatment principle is to tonify spleen qi and yang and warm the interior with herbs such as ginseng (ren shen), *Astragalus* (huang qi), ginger (gan jiang), and black pepper (hu jiao).

Spleen Qi Collapse or Spleen Qi Sinking: Since spleen qi supports the organs with its uplifting energy, this aspect of deficient qi is associated with a prolapse (sagging) and a sensation of bearing down in the internal organs. Some organs affected are the stomach, transverse colon, uterus, and rectum. Hemorrhoids are also a condition of spleen qi collapse. In some cases, miscarriages can occur from lack of qi to "hold things up," or retain the fetus with "upward" force. Treatment is to "raise the middle qi" with formulas such as Bu Zhong Yi Qi Tang ("Decoction to Tonify the Middle Burner and Raise the Vital Energy"). This formula contains herbs such as ginseng (ren shen) and *Astragalus* (huang qi) to build the spleen qi, along with herbs that have an uplifting energy such as *Bupleurum* (chai hu) and *Cimicifuga* (sheng ma).

Spleen Not Controlling the Blood: Another function of spleen qi is to keep blood flowing within the vessels. When this function is disturbed, symptoms of spleen qi deficiency occur along with bleeding under the skin (easy bruising), excessive menstrual bleeding, nosebleeds, and blood in the urine or stools. Since this bleeding is due to deficiency, the color of the blood is often lighter than might occur in excess bleeding disorders such as heat in the blood. Some of the Western disease patterns that could fall into this pattern are any chronic bleeding diseases, hemophilia, bleeding hemorrhoids, bruising from vitamin deficiency, and periodontal disease. The treatment is to tonify spleen qi and tonify blood. The classic formula for this purpose, Eight Treasure Decoction (Ba Zhen Tang), combines the standard formulas for qi and blood tonification.

Cold and Damp Surrounding the Spleen: This excess pattern arises when the dampness pernicious influence overwhelms the spleen. Symptoms include abdominal fullness and bloating, nausea, vomiting, watery stool, lack of thirst, sticky sensation and sweet taste in the mouth, dizziness, heavy feelings in the body, and a thick, greasy coat on the tongue. Some corresponding Western conditions are stomach "flu," chronic gastritis, chronic colitis, ulcers, and hepatitis. The treatment involves the use of fragrant herbs that "penetrate the dampness and wake up the spleen," such as patchouli (huo xiang).

Damp Heat in the Spleen: In this excess disharmony condition, the dampness symptoms combine with those of heat. They are: jaundice, yellow eyes, bitter taste in the mouth, nausea, vomiting, dislike of greasy food, burning urine and diarrhea, abdominal pain, bloating, and mouth sores. Some Western diagnoses are hepatitis, gallbladder disease, and acute gastroenteritis. The treatment principle is to clear damp heat with herbs such as *Coptis* (huang lian) and *Artemisia* (yin chen hao).

HEAT SYNDROMES

The heart governs the blood and vessels and is the seat of the mind and spirit. Disorders of the heart tend to involve emotional and mental disturbances as well as some circulatory conditions such as cold hands and feet. Generally, external pernicious influences don't affect the heart directly; instead, they typically attack the pericardium, the sac around the heart known in Chinese medicine as the "heart protector." In almost all disharmonies of the heart, palpitations are a key symptom. This pounding of the heart occurs in both excess and deficiency patterns.

Heart Qi Deficiency: Palpitations are the key symptom in this deficiency pattern. Other symptoms are spontaneous sweating, physical and mental fatigue, depression, pale face, and a weak pulse, especially in the heart area on the left wrist. This pattern can correspond to chronic fatigue, neurasthenia (chronic mental and physical weakness), or heart disease involving the muscle, valves, or vessels. The treatment principle for this deficiency is to tonify heart qi with standard qi tonics such as ginseng (ren shen), along with herbs that act specifically on the heart, such as *Schizandra* (wu wei zi) and *Biota* (bai zi ren).

Heart Yang Deficiency: This syndrome has all the symptoms of heart qi deficiency with the addition of cold symptoms: feeling cold in the limbs or entire body; purple face, tongue, and lips due to cold stagnating the circulation; and a slow, choppy, and intermittent pulse. A deeper, more serious condition than qi deficiency, heart yang deficiency typically corresponds to a Western diagnosis of true heart disease. The treatment is to tonify heart yang with moxibustion and herbs such as ginseng (ren shen) and aconite (fu zi). Note: Aconite is a highly toxic herb, and it should only be used in a formula prepared and supervised by a qualified practitioner of traditional Chinese medicine.

Heart Yang Collapse: A more severe version of heart yang deficiency, heart yang collapse produces all the symptoms of qi and yang deficiency plus copious cold sweats, extreme cold in the limbs, very weak breathing, a minute pulse, and abnormal shen that precedes a comatose state. Corresponding Western diagnoses are shock or heart attack, so this syndrome requires hospitalization. In China, the person receives herbal treatment while hospitalized. Typical treatment is an intravenous drip of *Salvia* (dan shen) and oral doses of ginseng (ren shen) and aconite (fu zi).

Heart Blood Deficiency: This pattern of deficiency involving the blood produces symptoms of palpitations, fearfulness and a propensity to be easily startled, insomnia, excessive dreams while asleep, mental restlessness, forgetfulness, dizziness, pale face and tongue, and a thin, small pulse. The insomnia is due to an insufficient amount of blood to provide a calm foundation for the spirit. Possibly corresponding to anemia or emotional imbalances, this deficiency syndrome is treated by tonifying heart blood with herbs such as *Angelica sinensis* (dang gui) and longan fruit (long yan rou).

Heart Yin Deficiency: This syndrome of deficiency heat produces red cheeks, night sweats, "five palm heat," dry mouth, thirst for small amounts of water, mental restlessness, insomnia, palpitations, low-grade fever, forgetfulness, excessive dreaming, red tongue with little or no coat, and a small, rapid pulse. A person with this deficiency has difficulty remaining asleep—the heat condition wakes them. Because the heart is the seat of the spirit, an insufficiency of calming, nurturing yin or blood in the heart results in agitation.

Hypertension and hyperthyroidism can match this pattern, which is treated with herbs that clear heat and tonify heart yin such as Emperor's Teapills (Tian Wang Bu Xin Dan).

Heart Fire Uprising: This excess heat pattern includes symptoms like a red face, dry mouth with a desire for lots of water, a red tip and prickles on the tongue with possible ulcers and pain, bitter taste in the mouth, burning urine, mental restlessness, insomnia, and a full, rapid pulse. Excess heat signs are stronger than those of heat due to yin deficiency. Some corresponding Western conditions are urinary tract infection, high blood pressure, or tongue infection. The treatment aims to clear heat and calm the spirit with acupuncture and herbs such as lotus seed sprouts (lian zi xin) and *Coptis* (huang lian).

Heart Blood Stagnation: This serious heart condition has symptoms of a sharp, stabbing pain in the heart area, pain that can radiate up the arm, purple face and tongue, fatigue, palpitations, and a choppy, wiry, or intermittent pulse. It sometimes occurs with heart yang or qi deficiency and includes the symptoms common to these patterns. Corresponding Western diseases are angina pectoris, coronary arteriosclerosis, or pericarditis—all requiring intensive medical intervention. Treatment involves regulating the qi and vitalizing the blood with circulatory stimulants such as *Salvia* (dan shen) and *Panax pseudoginseng* (san qi).

Hot Phlegm Confusing the Heart: This excess condition is characterized by excess heat causing a red face and eyes, irrational and possibly violent behavior, nonstop loud talking, anger, a red tongue with a greasy yellow coat, and a rapid, slippery pulse. It corresponds to the Western diagnoses of mental illness, mania, or encephalitis. The treatment for hot phlegm confusing the heart is to calm the spirit and clear heat and phlegm with acupuncture and herbs such as *Coptis* (huang lian) and *Borneol* (bing pian).

Phlegm Misting the Heart Opening: In this condition, which is related to the above syndrome but with less heat, symptoms include a pale tongue with a white coating, mental confusion, difficulty speaking (muttering to oneself, drooling), the sound of phlegm in the throat, and possible loss of consciousness. Some corresponding Western diseases are stroke, epilepsy, mental retardation, or mental illness. The treatment principle is to clear the phlegm and revive the consciousness with scalp acupuncture and herbs that resolve phlegm and wake up the spirit, such as *Calamus* (shi chang pu).

PERICARDIUM SYNDROMES

The pericardium is considered the sixth yin organ, but its functions are typically linked with the heart. The shield between the heart and the exterior, the pericardium protects the heart from the invasion of external pathogenic factors. Its main syndrome is known as "heat crushing the pericardium," which is characterized by a high fever, mental confusion, convulsions, and, possibly, coma. This pattern can appear in acute febrile diseases with a high fever, such as encephalitis or pericarditis, where the sudden high temperature affects the consciousness. Treatment includes the use of acupuncture points on the pericardium meridian, along with herbs that clear excess heat, such as tree peony root (mu dan pi).

LIVER SYNDROMES

Imbalances of the liver are seen commonly in clinical practice, since the stress and toxicity of modern life (poor diet, chemicals in our food and environment, stress, overwork, etc.) take a toll on this organ. Since the liver plays the central role in the smooth flow of qi and emotion in the body, disharmony of the liver can affect any of the other organs. Typically, disorders of the menstrual cycle or stress-related ailments indicate a problem with the liver.

Liver Qi Stagnation: This is one of the most common diagnoses in traditional Chinese medicine. When the qi of the liver is stuck, symptoms of frustration, irritability, depression, anxiety, fullness in the chest, menstrual disorders, and indigestion can occur. This excess condition can also arise in a person who has experienced long-term depression or frustrations, creating a vicious cycle of cause and effect. Some Western conditions that fit this pattern are premenstrual syndrome, depression, hepatitis, or chronic fatigue. Treatment with acupuncture often has an immediate effect in relieving the symptoms. A classic formula known as Xiao Yao Wan ("Free and Easy Wanderer Pills") is also very effective in rectifying this liver syndrome.

Liver Fire Uprising: This excess heat pattern mainly affects the upper body, since heat rises naturally. The entire face is red, with additional signs and symptoms of red eyes, anger, headache, ringing in the ears (tinnitus), bitter taste in the mouth, insomnia, constipation, dark urine, red tongue with a yellow coat, and a full, rapid pulse. The condition can arise from long-term stagnation of qi due to anger, alcoholism, or chronic liver imbalances that develop into heat patterns. Some corresponding Western diagnoses are hypertension, alcoholism, hyperthyroidism, acute hepatitis, gallbladder infection, ear infection, and conjunctivitis. Treatment involves clearing heat and regulating the liver with acupuncture and herbal formulas such as Long Dan Xie Gan Wan.

Liver and Gallbladder Damp Heat: When dampness accumulates in the body and combines with heat in the liver and gallbladder, this excess syndrome develops. Its symptoms are jaundice and dark urine, which are caused by a stagnation of yellow bile that backs up and is excreted through the skin and urine. Additional symptoms include a lack of appetite, an aversion to greasy food, digestive problems, bitter taste in the mouth, nausea, vomiting, burning diarrhea, a red tongue with a thick, greasy yellow coat, and a slippery, rapid pulse. In Western medicine, most of these symptoms are typical of acute hepatitis or gallbladder infections, but this pattern can also correspond to herpes, vaginal discharges, testicular pain, and eczema. The treatment principle is to clear heat and drain dampness with herbs such as rhubarb root (da huang), gentian (long dan cao), and *Artemisia* (yin chen hao).

Liver Wind Moving Internally: Since the liver is in charge of the smooth flow of qi, any abnormal body movements are typically related to liver imbalances due to wind. This internal wind is considered an excess pattern, but it can arise from a variety of causes, such as blood deficiency, excess heat, or liver yin deficiency. The cardinal symptoms involve abnormal movements such as shaking, spasms, tics, rigidity, and convulsions. Dizziness, headache, and difficulty in speaking may also occur. The tongue and pulse signs depend on which underlying pattern has caused the stirring of wind, but the pulse is usually wiry, a typical sign of liver imbalance. This pattern is seen in stroke patients and those with Parkinson disease and cases of seizures associated with a high fever, tetanus, and hypertension. Acupuncture can be a very effective treatment, as are herbs that clear liver wind and heat, such as *Gastrodia* (tian ma), *Uncaria* (gou teng), and *Chrysanthemum* (jua hua). If the problem is caused by depletion, the underlying deficiency must be tonified. For example, if wind is due to deficient liver yin, treatment must both tonify the liver yin and subdue the wind.

Cold Stagnation in the Liver Channel: The liver meridian encircles the genital area, so localized disorders in the reproductive organs are often traced to a blockage in that meridian. This syndrome is characterized by pain in the groin, lower abdomen, and testicles and is relieved by application of heat. This pattern typically corresponds to a hernia but may also be present in cold-type menstrual disorders and infertility. Treatment involves warming with moxa and using herbs that regulate qi and warm the liver meridian, such as *Galangal* (gao liang jiang) and lychee seed (li zhi he).

Liver Blood Deficiency: This syndrome has the typical symptoms of blood deficiency: pale face and tongue, dizziness, dry skin, and thin pulse. The condition of the eyes and nails are clues to the state of the liver, so symptoms may include pale, cracked nails, blurred vision, itchy eyes, night blindness, and visual distortions such as spots and floaters. Menstrual flow may be scanty, and lack of nourishment to the tendons from liver blood deficiency can lead to pain, numbness, or cramping. Possible Western diagnoses are anemia, malnutrition, hypertension, menstrual disorders, and eye problems. Treatment involves tonifying the blood with blood tonics such as *Angelica sinensis* (dang gui), cooked *Rehmannia* (shu di huang), and *Polygonum multiflorum* (he shou wu), along with herbs that specifically nourish the liver such as *Lycium* fruit (gou qi zi).

Liver Yin Deficiency: This syndrome exhibits the usual signs of "five palm heat": red cheeks, night sweats, red tongue with no coat, and a thin, rapid pulse. Additional symptoms specific to the liver are dizziness, irritability, and dry, irritated eyes. Treatment involves tonifying liver yin and clearing heat with formulas such as *Chrysanthemum*, *Lycium*, and *Rehmannia* Pills (Qi Ju Di Huang Wan).

Liver Yang Rising: If liver yin deficiency continues without treatment, the deficiency heat rises to the head. Known as liver yang rising, it produces additional symptoms of headache and anger. It is an intermediate syndrome—more severe than a simple yin deficiency but less severe than liver fire. Some Western diagnoses are anemia, chronic hepatitis, hypertension, eye problems, menopause, and menstrual disorders. Treatment involves sedating the excess liver yang with formulas such as Gastrodia and Uncaria Combination (Tian Ma Gou Teng Yin). If the yang rising symptoms are especially severe, heavy herbs that settle yang, such as oyster shell (mu li), are added.

KIDNEY SYNDROMES

Since the kidneys are the source of yin and yang for the entire body, a kidney imbalance can have an effect anywhere in the body. They are the storage site for the essence, the substance responsible for growth, fertility, and vitality, so the kidneys are only subject to syndromes of deficiency. Patterns of deficient qi, yin, or yang are often traced to a corresponding syndrome of deficiency within the kidneys; similarly, a long-term depletion in any organ eventually depletes the kidneys.

Kidney Yang Deficiency: The kidney yang is the source of metabolic fire (the heat needed for digestion and other bodily functions) for the entire body. When kidney yang is depleted, symptoms are cold hands and feet, frequent urination with clear urine or water retention and edema, night urination, pallor, pain in the lower back and knees, low sex drive, apathy, and an aversion to cold environments. This chronic condition can correspond to the Western conditions of nephritis, hypothyroidism, adrenal insufficiency, chronic low back pain, depression, and sexual dysfunction. Treatment involves tonifying the "life-gate fire" by applying heat from moxibustion at a point below the second lumbar vertebra. The standard herb formula is Rehmannia Eight (Ba Wei Di Huang Wan), which contains herbs that nourish the kidneys along with hot metabolic stimulants such as cinnamon bark (rou gui) and aconite (fu zi).

Kidney Yang Deficiency with Dirty Water Flooding: This syndrome exhibits all the above symptoms of yang deficiency, but in this case the lack of yang leads to a debility in fluid transformation (fluids don't move to their proper locations; instead, they collect in organs or limbs). The specific symptoms elated to this metabolic failure include edema in the lower body, abdominal fullness, nausea, difficulty breathing, cough or asthma with thin mucus, and small amounts of clear urine. This syndrome can correspond to congestive heart failure or nephritis. Treatment consists of tonifying kidney yang as above, with the addition of diuretic herbs such as *Plantago* seeds (che qian zi) and ginger root skin (sheng jiang pi).

Kidney Yin Deficiency: This condition of deficiency heat is due to a depletion of the yin. Typical yin deficiency signs of red cheeks, night sweats, "five palm heat," dry mouth, a red tongue with little or no coat, and a thin, rapid pulse occur. In addition, depletion symptoms specific to the kidneys occur, such as concentrated urine, nocturnal emissions of semen, premature ejaculation, overactive sex drive, vertigo, ringing in the ears, insomnia, and sore low back and knees. This pattern might match Western diagnoses of lumbago, hypertension, diabetes, hyperthyroidism, and psychological or emotional disorders. The standard base formula for all varieties of kidney yin deficiency is Rehmannia Teapills (Liu Wei Di Huang Wan).

Kidney Essence (Jing) Deficiency: The kidney essence is responsible for growth, development, and reproduction. Children with this deficiency may exhibit late closure of the soft spots in the skull, slow growth, late development of speech and walking, or mental retardation. Adults may experience premature aging, fragile bones, loss of teeth and hair, infertility, and poor memory. In children, the syndrome is entirely genetic; in adults the pattern arises from old age or "burning the candle at both ends." Treatment consists of tonifying kidney yin and yang; the balance of warm and cold herbs is tailored to fit the individual situation. In addition, herbs are used that specifically strengthen the essence, such as privet fruit (nu zhen zi) and *Cuscuta* (tu si zi).

SMALL INTESTINE SYNDROMES

The small intestine's functions are to separate food and fluids into essential and waste components. A yang organ, its patterns of disharmony are usually related to a dysfunction in a yin organ such as the heart or spleen.

Small Intestine Deficient and Cold: This pattern can arise in a deficiency of spleen yang. Symptoms include pain around the navel that is relieved with pressure and heat, watery diarrhea or loose stools, frequent clear urination, and a gurgling sound in the abdomen. The tongue is pale with a white coat, and the pulse is deep, empty, and slow. Some corresponding Western conditions are infections with the Candida organism, food allergies, enteritis, chronic dysentery, or stress-related digestive disorders. Treatment involves tonifying spleen yang with moxibustion and warm, strengthening herbs such as ginseng (ren shen) and ginger (gan jiang).

Small Intestine Excess Heat: Excess heat in the heart can be transferred to the small intestine, since the two organs are paired in a yin/yang relationship. When this occurs, the symptoms include frequent dark burning urine, thirst, a red tip on the tongue, mental restlessness, and a rapid, full pulse. Although the cause is often emotional hyperactivity, the excess heat shows up in the urine in a typical Western diagnosis of urinary tract infection. The treatment principle is to clear heat from the heart and small intestine with acupuncture and herbs such as *Lophatherum* (dan zhu ye) and lotus sprout (lian zi xin).

Small Intestine Qi Pain: Often associated with stagnant liver qi, this pattern exhibits distention and pain in the lower abdomen that feels worse when pressure is applied, distention and pain in the groin, gurgling sounds in the abdominal area, pain relief after passing gas, a pale tongue with a thin, white coat, and a deep, wiry pulse. Corresponding Western conditions might be hernia of the small intestine, colitis, food allergies, and enteritis. Since it is a disorder of stagnant qi, acupuncture and stress reduction are particularly helpful to treat it. Herbal therapy includes herbs to regulate qi, such as *Bupleurum* (chai hu), white peony root (bai shao), and *Cyperus* (xiang fu).

LARGE INTESTINE SYNDROMES

The large intestine has the same functions in traditional Chinese medicine as it does in Western physiology: receiving food from the small intestine, separating the fluids, and passing on the remainder as waste. Dysfunctions of the large intestine typically involve a disruption in one of these activities, often due to poor dietary habits.

Large Intestine Excess Heat: This excess syndrome is characterized by constipation, a bloated, painful abdomen, fever, explosive burning diarrhea with a bad smell, concentrated urine, thirst, a red tongue with a thick yellow coat, and a full, rapid pulse. It is associated with acute bacterial dysentery or any serious infection. Treatment involves clearing the excess heat from the large intestine with cooling purgative herbs such as rhubarb (da huang) and *Mirabilite* (mang xiao).

Large Intestine Damp Heat: This pattern is similar to the excess heat syndrome described above, with the addition of the influence of dampness, which makes recovery slower than with simple excess heat. The dampness also creates the additional symptoms of fatigue, a sensation of not being finished when defecating, blood or pus in the stools, intermittent fever, a slippery pulse, and a greasy yellow tongue coating. This pattern corresponds to acute amoebic dysentery or hemorrhoids and is treated with herbs that clear the dampness and heat from the large intestine, such as *Coptis* (huang lian) and *Pulsatilla* (bai tou weng).

Large Intestine Closed and Knotted: This excess pattern has symptoms of abdominal bloating with pain that gets worse when pressure is applied, constipation, nausea, vomiting, deep, full pulse, and a greasy, thick white coat on the tongue. It is seen in intestinal blockages due to a hernia or scar tissue and is often seen in children. Typically, surgery is required. If the blockage is only partial, acupuncture and strong purgative herbs such as *Croton* (ba dou) can alleviate the symptoms.

Heat Stagnation in the Large Intestine: This excess pattern, which combines excess heat with qi and blood stagnation, causes sharp, fixed abdominal pain that worsens when pressure is applied, bloating, constipation or diarrhea, vomiting, fever, a deep-red tongue with a thick yellow dry coat, and a full, wiry, rapid pulse. Possible Western diagnoses are appendicitis, diverticulitis, and dysentery.

This is a serious condition, and proper medical intervention is essential. An acupuncture point on the leg known as Lanwei is specific for appendicitis. Since this condition can be caused by hardened feces blocking the appendix, stimulating this point could dislodge the blockage, explaining this point's effectiveness in treating early-stage appendicitis. Treatment includes cooling, purgative herbs such as rhubarb root (da huang) and herbs such as tree peony root (mu dan pi) to move stagnant qi and blood.

Large Intestine Fluid Deficiency: The fluid deficiency in this syndrome can arise from old age, dehydration after an illness, delivery of a baby, or chronic infections. The symptoms are chronic constipation, dry mouth, dry stools, small and rapid pulse, and a dry, red, and cracked tongue. The treatment principle for this syndrome is to clear heat and moisten the intestines with herbs such as *Cannabis* seeds (huo ma ren) and *Rehmannia* root (sheng di huang).

Large Intestine Deficient and Cold: Most often a result of spleen yang deficiency, this pattern has symptoms of watery diarrhea without a strong smell, abdominal pain relieved by pressure and warmth, gurgling abdominal sounds, a worsening of symptoms after eating cold food, deep weak pulse, and a pale, swollen tongue with teeth marks. Treatment includes herbs that tonify spleen yang, such as dried ginger (gan jiang), as well as moxibustion to points on the abdomen.

STOMACH SYNDROMES

All the stomach's functions involve breaking down food, so stomach disorders typically include digestive disturbances. Since the stomach and spleen are intimately related in a yin/yang polarity, imbalances in one organ often affect the other.

Stomach Fire: This syndrome of internal excess heat is characterized by a burning pain in the upper abdominal area, excessive hunger even after eating, thirst, bad breath, canker sores in the mouth, pain and bleeding in the gums, nausea, vomiting, red tongue with a thick, dry yellow coat, and a strong, rapid pulse. Some parallel Western diagnoses might be gastric ulcer or stomatitis, and treatment involves herbs that clear stomach fire, such as *Coptis* (huang lian).

Food Stagnation: This excess syndrome, usually due to overeating, can have either cold or heat signs. Symptoms include a lack of appetite, a full, bloated feeling in the stomach, nausea, vomiting, bad breath, and acid belching. Treatment of food stagnation includes herbs that move qi in the stomach, such as green tangerine peel (qing pi), along with herbs that relieve the food stagnation itself. If the person has overindulged in fatty foods, the herb of choice is hawthorn berries (shan zha); when the syndrome results from overeating of grains, barley sprouts (mai ya) are preferred.

Stomach Yin Deficiency: Symptoms of this deficiency syndrome include a lack of appetite, thirst with an inability to drink more than a few sips, dry mouth and lips, dry stools, a thin, rapid pulse, and a red tongue with no coat, especially in the center. Since the stomach yin is the source of the tongue coat, its corresponding area in the middle of the tongue appears especially peeled. This syndrome can match a Western diagnosis of chronic gastric ulcer or chronic gastritis. The herbal treatment focuses on tonifying stomach yin with herbs such as *Dendrobium* (shi hu) and *Ophiopogon* (mai men dong).

Stomach Deficient and Cold: A pattern of deficiency typically involving the spleen, it has symptoms of "dirty water stagnation": When the person moves, it is possible to hear liquids splashing. Other symptoms of this pattern are dull pains in the stomach area that are relieved by pressure and warmth, excessive sputum in the mouth, fatigue, bloating, and diarrhea. The pulse is slow, weak, slippery, and deficient, while the tongue is pale with a greasy white coat. This pattern of deficiency could possibly correspond to a Western diagnosis of food allergies, infection with the Candida organism, or chronic gastroenteritis. Moxibustion to points on the abdomen is quite helpful in treating a cold disorder such as this. Herbal therapy includes use of herbs that are warming to the stomach such as ginger (gan jiang), tonics such as ginseng (ren shen), and dampness-draining herbs such as *Poria* (fu ling).

GALLBLADDER SYNDROMES

The gallbladder is related to the liver, both in a yin/yang relationship and physical proximity. The liver produces bile, while the gallbladder stores and secretes it. Since a strong gallbladder helps a person be assertive and decisive, imbalances in the organ can lead to indecision and timidity.

Phlegm Confusing the Gallbladder: When the gallbladder is weak and under the influence of dampness, this syndrome can develop. Its symptoms are dizziness, blurry vision, nausea, being easily startled, indecisiveness, frightening dreams, vomiting with a bitter taste, dull pain or distention in the rib area, a pale, puffy tongue with a greasy white coating, and a slippery, wiry pulse. Corresponding Western conditions might include emotional or psychological disorders, hypertension (especially in people who are overweight), and menopausal symptoms. Treatment for this syndrome includes herbal formulas that calm the spirit and clear phlegm from the gallbladder, such as Gallbladder Warming Decoction (Wen Dan Tang).

URINARY BLADDER SYNDROMES

The urinary bladder performs the functions of receiving waste water from the kidneys and excreting it from the body. It is paired in a yin/yang relationship with the kidneys, so a deficiency in the urinary bladder is typically related to a deficiency in the kidneys. The kidneys have no excess syndromes, so any excess pattern in the urinary tract is diagnosed as a urinary bladder disharmony.

Urinary Bladder Damp Heat: This excess pattern has symptoms of pain and distention in the lower abdomen, frequent urination that is burning and produces dark urine, possible stones or blood in the urine, low back pain, and a rapid, slippery pulse. The tongue is red with a thick, greasy yellow coating, especially in the back area of the tongue, which corresponds to the lower burner. Some possible corresponding Western diagnoses are urinary tract infection, urinary tract stones, or prostate disorders. The treatment principle is to clear lower burner damp heat with herbs such as *Dianthus* (qu mai), *Phellodendron* (huang bai), and *Andrographis* (chuan xin lian).

Urinary Bladder Deficient and Cold: If the kidney qi or yang is depleted, this deficiency syndrome can occur in the bladder. Symptoms are frequent urination that is clear and copious, occasional difficulty in urinating, inability to hold in the urine, bed-wetting, feelings of cold and pain in the lower abdomen or lower back, a deep, weak pulse, and a pale, moist, puffy tongue with a thin white coat. It can be diagnosed as a chronic urinary tract infection or prostate disorder, and treatment involves moxibustion on the lower abdomen. Herbal therapy focuses on tonifying kidney yang with herbs such as *Rehmannia* (shu di huang), Aconite (fu zi), and cinnamon bark (rou gui).

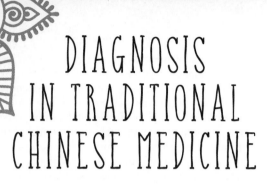

DIAGNOSIS IN TRADITIONAL CHINESE MEDICINE

LOOKING

The Face: An experienced practitioner often develops an initial idea of a patient's health just by observing him or her walking into the office. Inspecting the quality of the spirit (shen) is an important aspect of this first impression, since the shen gives a good indication of the overall vitality of a person. The shen especially shows in the eyes: An ancient maxim states, "If there is shen, there is life." A person with healthy shen has a gleam or sparkle of life in the eyes. The face is bright with some color, breathing is regular, and movements and speech are normal and logical. A person with unhealthy spirit has dim eyes with a vacant look. The face is dull with no shine; breathing is slow, weak, or irregular; movements appear abnormal or unusual; and speech is illogical or the voice is at an inappropriate volume.

Changes in facial skin color can provide the traditional Chinese medicine practitioner with a number of diagnostic clues. A bright (shiny), white face can indicate deficiency of qi or a cold condition, while a dull, pale face with no shine is a sign of blood deficiency. Redness in the face indicates heat: If the entire face is red, it is a sign of excess heat, while red cheeks alone are a sign of deficiency heat. A bright yellow skin tone can indicate damp heat, while pale yellow is a sign of damp cold due to deficiency. Finally, areas of black usually indicate kidney deficiency. The location of color on the face also has diagnostic significance as in the example of kidney deficiency: The black appears below the eyes and is often seen in people who don't get enough sleep or push themselves too hard, both practices that deplete the kidneys of qi, yin, and yang. Another example of the importance of the location of color is when it appears on the tip of the nose, an area affected by the spleen. Alcoholics often have redness in this area due to damp heat in the spleen caused by the heat generated in that organ by alcohol.

The Body: A lot of information can also be accumulated by looking at the overall physique. Overweight people have a tendency toward dampness or phlegm, while thin people are inclined to be yin deficient. A person with internal heat may be scantily clad in the winter, while a person with internal cold might wear a sweater in the summer. Somebody who is active and energetic tends to experience yang syndromes, while yin syndromes are more common in quiet, sedentary people. Faded, sparse, and dry hair indicates weak kidney qi or blood, while lustrous, thick, and shiny hair is a sign of strong kidney qi and sufficient blood. Finally, the lips can tell a lot about the condition of the body. Bright red lips can indicate heat, pale lips can be a sign of qi or blood deficiency, and blue lips can be due to cold or blood stagnation. Dry and cracked lips are a sign of depleted body fluids, and twitching lips are an indication of liver wind.

The Tongue: The most important and richest source of visual diagnostic information is the tongue. Entire books have been written to illustrate the amount of information that can be garnered simply by carefully observing the tongue. The surface of the tongue is divided into areas that correspond to the organs. The tip of the tongue corresponds to the heart, while the entire front area applies to the lungs. The middle area reflects the condition of the stomach and spleen, while the sides of the tongue are related to the liver and gallbladder. Finally, the back of the tongue corresponds to the lower burner, which includes the kidneys, the urinary bladder, and the large intestine. These assigned areas reveal a wealth of information, and they repeatedly prove accurate when applied to clinical practice.

The colors of the tongue body and coating also enhance the picture. When the body of the tongue is much redder than normal, it is a sign of excess heat, while a slightly redder tongue body is a sign of deficiency heat. A pale tongue body indicates a syndrome of deficiency or cold. A purple tongue can indicate qi or blood stagnation, while a blue-tinged tongue indicates stagnation and severe deficiency of qi and blood. The consistency and shape of the tongue are also significant. A puffy tongue with teeth marks on the sides is seen in a person with deficient qi, while a puffy tongue that appears wet indicates deficient yang. A shriveled, atrophied tongue is seen in deficient conditions; this sign appears sometimes in cancer patients. Finally, cracking in the tongue body occurs when body fluids have been depleted due to heat or yin deficiency.

The movements of the tongue also tell their own story. When the tongue shakes, it is a sign of deficiency or liver wind. (Of course, it can also indicate nervousness.) When a person has difficulty sticking the tongue out, it can indicate deficient qi, blood, or yin. When the tongue is turned to one side, as in stroke patients, it is a sign of internal wind or phlegm blocking the meridians. Finally, a person who leaves his tongue out, or whose tongue moves in and out, has heat in the heart.

Another important aspect of diagnosis through observation of the tongue is the appearance of the coating on the tongue. In a healthy person, the coating is thin, moist, and white. A change in the coating's color or distribution indicates some sort of pathologic process occurring in the internal organs; for example, if there is heat in the stomach, that area of the tongue will have a yellow coating. A thick coating is related to excess conditions, while a thin coating is seen in deficiency. With yin deficiency, there is little or no coating, since the tongue coating is created by the stomach yin. An excessively moist coating is a sign of excess fluids and occurs when yang is insufficient to transform fluids (in other words, if yang is weak, fluids accumulate). A dry coating indicates fluid deficiency or dehydration; a greasy coating indicates dampness; and a patchy coating occurs when phlegm blocks the acupuncture meridians.

The color of the tongue coating can tell a lot about the nature and progress of a disease. Often, an acupuncturist requests that patients avoid brushing the tongue before an office visit, since it can take a few hours for the coating to reappear. Similarly, foods that discolor the tongue should also be avoided before an appointment, since they can make it difficult or impossible for a practitioner to read the true coating color. Although a white tongue coating is normal, it can also appear in external conditions, as well as conditions of cold or deficiency. A yellow tongue coating is always a sign of heat; as the heat increases, the intensity of the color also increases. A gray or black tongue coating can appear in conditions of extreme heat or cold, depending on the other symptoms. The progress of a disease can actually be monitored by observing the tongue over the course of an illness. A person with a high fever might have a thick yellow coating; as the fever subsides, the coating becomes more white as the excess heat leaves the body.

There are actually many more sophisticated visual diagnostic cues, but they are beyond the scope of this book. However, the above descriptions illustrate that a wealth of information is available to the observant practitioner before hearing a single word of complaint from a patient.

LISTENING AND SMELLING

Listening and smelling are two additional ways that the practitioner can garner information about a patient. The two diagnostic tools are grouped together because the same Chinese word is used for both of them. In this diagnostic area, the practitioner listens to the various sounds emanating from the patient and pays attention to any unusual smells. A wealth of information can be gleaned from these perceptions, and they give the physician some clues to pursue later on during the initial interview.

LISTENING

Speaking: A person under attack by an external pathogen speaks softly at first, with the voice gradually becoming louder. With an internal deficiency, the voice gets softer over time due to a lack of energy. People with cold syndromes tend to be quiet, while heat syndromes are associated with excessive talking. It is the nature of cold to slow functions and movement, while heat speeds them up. A person with an excess condition tends to have a loud, strong voice, while a soft, weak voice is associated with deficiency patterns. Repeated sighing is often a sign of liver qi stagnation; it is an attempt by the body to release pent-up emotion while expanding the chest muscles that tighten due to the stagnation.

Breathing: Weak and shallow breathing that is difficult to hear is associated with deficiency, especially of the lungs and kidneys. Loud and heavy breathing indicates an excess condition that constricts the air passages. The source of asthmatic wheezing can also be differentiated by its sounds. In a deficiency pattern, the sound is soft and the patient experiences difficulty inhaling due to the kidneys' inability to "grasp the qi." In a lung excess syndrome, the wheezing is coarse and loud and the patient has difficulty exhaling. A loud cough is a sign of excess, while a weak, slow cough is due to deficiency. A dry, hacking sound can indicate dryness or yin deficiency, while gurgling sounds are a sign of phlegm.

Gastrointestinal Signs: Vomiting due to an excess condition is loud and strong, while a deficiency condition causes vomiting that is weak and painful. Hiccups are known as "rebellious stomach qi" in traditional Chinese diagnosis. If they are due to excess, the sound is loud and short, while deficiency hiccups have a weak sound and last longer. If hiccups show up in an illness after a few days, it is an indication of a collapse of stomach qi. Loud belching is a sign of excess; if there is heat, a sour smell accompanies the belching. Deficiency belching has a softer sound with no sour smell.

SMELLING

In general, strong smells are due to heat, while a lack of aroma is a sign of cold. This applies to the breath, urine, stools, vomit, sweat, and any discharges. Some specific smells are linked to organs; for example, a sweet smell is linked to the spleen, a urine-like smell is associated with a kidney problem, and a smell like rotten apples is a sign of diabetes ("wasting and thirsting syndrome").

ASKING

This is an exceptionally important aspect of diagnosis, for Western as well as traditional Chinese practitioners. When interviewing the patient, the traditional Chinese practitioner accumulates enough information to formulate a diagnosis based on the condition of the internal organs, pernicious influences, and vital substances. The traditional Chinese practitioner also delves further into information that he or she uncovered while "looking, listening, and smelling." In addition, the practitioner attempts to get an accurate picture of the person's past medical history, lifestyle, and present area of complaint, gradually building a complete diagnostic picture.

CHILLS AND FEVER

It is important to remember that these terms refer more to the patient's perceptions of cold or heat, rather than an actual elevated body temperature or shivering. Chills and fever that occur simultaneously indicate an external condition: If the chills are worse than the fever, the condition is wind cold; if the fever is worse than the chills, it is wind heat. In either case, if the fever persists after the chills disappear, it is a sign that the condition has penetrated to the interior of the body. If the fever persists and is accompanied by sweating, thirst, and constipation, the interior heat has penetrated to the stomach and intestines, which is an even deeper level. A chronic low-grade fever can occur after an illness accompanied by a fever has "burned out the yin." This sort of fever can also be a sign of qi deficiency associated with a collapse of the body's immune system.

Feeling cold can be a symptom of either wind cold or yang deficiency. In wind cold, it can be difficult for a person to get warm, even when he or she is bundled up in warm clothes. Wind cold is an acute ailment of short duration, while yang deficiency is a long-term, chronic condition.

PERSPIRATION

Perspiration is regulated through the opening and closing of the pores, a function of the defensive qi (wei qi). When qi or yang deficiency occurs, the pores remain open due to weakness, and the person experiences spontaneous sweating during the day. This can occur even if the person has not become overheated. Sensations of heat in the evening with night sweats are considered a sign of yin deficiency. This condition is called "stealing sweats" because it steals fluids from the body like a thief in the night. In an external disorder, perspiration is an important indicator of the final diagnosis: With wind heat, the person perspires, while with wind cold, the pores are closed from cold, causing a lack of sweating. If sweating occurs with an external condition, and the person feels better afterward, it is a sign that the body has successfully expelled the pathogen. If sweating doesn't break the fever or make the person feel better, the pathogen is successfully fighting against the wei qi.

HEAD AND BODY

Headaches that have an acute onset with severe pain are usually due to an external pernicious influence, such as wind cold or wind heat. Milder, more chronic headache pain suggests an internal influence such as qi or blood deficiency. Severe, intermittent pain is likely due to liver fire, which rises up to the head, often from an outburst of anger. The location of the headache also has clinical significance, since it helps the physician select herbs and acupuncture meridians that run through the area of pain. For example, a frontal headache is considered a disorder of the stomach meridian. Treatment involves needling acupuncture points on that meridian and prescribing herbs with an affinity for that area of the body. Pain at the top or sides of the head is related to the liver and gallbladder, while pain at the back of the head is related to the bladder meridian.

Dizziness is another important diagnostic aspect associated with the head. If dizziness is due to qi deficiency, the symptoms are mild and get worse when the person is tired. Blood deficiency dizziness is also mild and gets worse when the person stands up suddenly. Dizziness from dampness is associated with a heavy feeling, which patients often describe as a "wet blanket wrapped around the head." Liver fire can create a severe form of dizziness in which the person loses balance as if on a rolling ship. If the head itself is shaking, it is a sign of internal wind moving.

Since many people turn to traditional Chinese medicine for the treatment of pain, this is often the first symptom mentioned to a practitioner. The practitioner can accumulate an abundance of information by asking about the location, severity, frequency, and causes of pain in the patient's body. Pain that comes and goes is due to wind or qi stagnation, while pain in a fixed location is a result of cold or blood stagnation. If pressure relieves the pain, it is a deficient type; pressure always makes excess type pain feel worse. Pain in specific areas of the body can also serve as a sign of problems in an internal organ. For example, pain in the rib area is a symptom of stagnation in the liver and gallbladder. Lower back pain is a cardinal sign of kidney deficiency: Since it is due to depletion, it gets worse after exertion. When low back pain is due to cold and dampness, a stagnant condition, it gets worse after rest.

EARS AND EYES

Since the kidneys open up into the ears, poor hearing or deafness is usually from kidney deficiency. Sudden deafness is usually due to heat and fire rising up to the ears, which is an excess condition. Similarly, ringing in the ears (tinnitus) is a sign of an excess condition if it comes on suddenly as a loud, high sound. Most often this is a condition of liver yang rising up to the head. Development of tinnitus over a long time is a sign of depletion of the kidneys. One diagnostic test is to press on the ears. If the sound gets stronger, it is due to excess; if it gets weaker, it is due to deficiency.

The eyes can also tell a lot about the patient. As previously mentioned, a practitioner looks into the eyes to assess the state of a person's shen (spirit) and thus acquire a general picture of the overall vitality and the potential for healing. Pain in the eyes can be due to liver fire or wind heat, while dry eyes can be caused by blood deficiency. Poor vision in general is associated with kidney jing or liver blood deficiency, as is night blindness. Itching in the eyes is a symptom of external wind or blood deficiency. Abnormal eye movement is a sign of internal wind.

STOOLS AND URINE

The stools and urine are important sources of information but may be signs overlooked by the patient. Stools that are sticky or cause burning with a strong smell are a sign of heat, while watery diarrhea with little smell is a sign of deficiency or cold. Damp heat causes frequent urges to defecate, but only a small amount is expelled each time. Stools that are watery with undigested food indicate spleen yang deficiency; if the same symptoms occur early in the morning ("cock's crow diarrhea"), it is due to kidney yang deficiency.

When constipation occurs, other diagnostic signs must be taken into account. If constipation accompanies dark urine, bad breath, and a yellow tongue coat, heat is the cause. Qi stagnation is the cause if the constipation occurs when the person is upset; qi deficiency is implicated if a person feels fatigued after a bowel movement. In blood or yin deficiency, the stools are exceptionally dry, making them difficult to pass.

Frequent passing of clear urine indicates kidney deficiency; if the urine is concentrated (dark yellow), it is a sign of heat. Bed-wetting can also occur in kidney deficiency; in children, the cause of the bed-wetting is usually emotional. Lack of urination can arise from very deficient kidneys or occur due to severe heat, blood stagnation, or a stone. Whatever its cause, lack of urination is a life-threatening condition, since the body can quickly become overwhelmed by its own toxins. In general, pale urine is a sign of cold, dark urine is a sign of heat, and cloudy urine is a sign of dampness. Sharp pain or blood in the urine can result from a stone or heat in the urinary bladder. Blood without pain could be a sign of cancer.

THIRST, APPETITE, AND TASTE

No desire for fluids at all is a sign of excess cold, while a desire for small amounts of hot liquids can indicate deficiency cold from yang depletion. A craving for large amounts of water is a sign of excess heat. If a person has a dry mouth and wants small amounts of water, it is a sign of deficiency heat due to depleted yin. If dampness is present, a person may want to drink but is unable to do so and may even vomit small amounts of water.

A person with an excessively strong appetite may have stomach heat; he or she might even eat a lot but remain thin. A person who has an appetite but no desire to eat could have stomach yin deficiency. In this case, the deficiency heat causes a false appetite, but the deficiency in stomach yin itself prevents true hunger. On the other hand, a complete lack of appetite indicates spleen qi deficiency; when the person does eat, he or she often feels bloated or tired afterward. When the appetite is low and the person has an aversion to oily foods, the cause could be damp heat in the liver and gallbladder.

Another set of diagnostic indicators unique to traditional Chinese medicine is the presence of various tastes in the mouth. For example, a bitter taste in the mouth indicates heat, usually in the heart, liver, or gallbladder. A sweet taste can occur with damp heat in the spleen, and a salty taste can arise from a deficiency in the kidneys. A sour taste is associated with heat in the liver or food stagnation in the stomach, while a complete lack of taste can occur with spleen qi deficiency.

SLEEP

A restful night's sleep depends on a healthy balance of yin and yang. The yin and blood are the aspects of the heart that provide a solid foundation for the mind and spirit. If yin and blood are deficient, yang will be out of control. Yang is fire and activity and is kept within normal ranges by cool and calm yin. When yin is deficient, it can't control yang, and too much heat and activity results, producing such symptoms as restlessness and insomnia. On the other hand, if qi or yang is insufficient, the person experiences an overabundance of yin, leading to fatigue and excessive sleepiness. A person who has difficulty falling asleep but then sleeps soundly may have a deficiency of heart blood. Difficulty staying asleep can be a sign of deficient heart yin: The deficiency heat disturbs sleep. Insomnia that is accompanied by a bitter taste in the mouth and angry dreams is associated with liver fire, while sleeplessness due to irritability and sexual dreams can be a result of heat due to kidney yin deficiency. A person who wakes up easily, is forgetful, and experiences heart palpitations can have a pattern of insufficient heart blood and spleen qi. In children, crying at night can often be due to heat in the heart or liver.

A practitioner also attempts to determine whether a person gets too much sleep, since this could be due to qi or yang deficiency. If the person claims his whole body feels heavy, especially when the weather is rainy, the excessive sleep is caused by dampness.

LIFESTYLE AND MEDICAL HISTORY

Many imbalances are due to the patient's lifestyle. It is very difficult to treat a case of cold dampness in the spleen successfully in a person who eats a quart of ice cream every day—no matter how much ginseng and ginger the person consumes. Ice cream is classified as a cold, damp food. On the other hand, the same person can assist the healing process by consuming hot soups containing ginger root and pepper. Foods are also strong medicines with their own hot or cold energies, and selecting the proper foods for a given body type or disease pattern is an important part of the healing process. Similarly, a person who walks around barefoot in the winter might complain about frequent colds. This person would be better off dressing in warm clothing, rather than trying to stimulate the immune system.

A complete medical history is just as important in traditional Chinese medicine as it is in Western medicine. Important clues might be uncovered that could shed light on the cause of current problems. It's important to note the use of any prescription medication, since a patient's symptoms could be due to side effects of these medications.

GYNECOLOGIC SIGNS AND SYMPTOMS

A female patient is always asked about her menstrual cycle, since it can provide abundant information about the condition of the internal organs and vital substances. A cycle that is longer than normal might be a sign of blood deficiency or cold stagnation, while a short cycle can occur with heat. A scanty menstrual flow with light-colored blood is associated with deficiency of qi and blood, while a strong flow with dark color can be a sign of excess heat. Cramping before the menstrual flow is a symptom of excess, while cramping after the flow begins is a sign of deficiency. Blood clots with sharp pains occur with blood stagnation. If there is no cycle at all, the primary causes are qi and blood deficiency or stagnation.

TOUCHING

The art of touch in traditional Chinese medicine is highly sophisticated and includes the palpation of areas of pain and diagnostic points and the reading of the patient's pulse. For example, an area of the body that feels hot to the touch is experiencing a heat condition, while a place that is cold to the touch is under the influence of cold or dampness. Tumors or swellings that are hard with a well-defined border are due to blood stagnation, while soft nodules with an indistinct border are a result of qi or phlegm stagnation.

Diagnostic points on each acupuncture meridian can be palpated to assess the condition of an internal organ. When there is an imbalance in the organ, the point is painful or has a flaccid feeling. For example, there are points on the back known as transporting points, each one corresponding to an internal organ. If an imbalance occurs in one of these organs, the transporting point for that organ might be tender or sore. The treatment would include needling that point in order to heal the organ that is associated with it. The Japanese have also developed a highly sophisticated system of abdominal palpation; entire books have been written on the subject.

By far, the most important form of palpation in Chinese medicine is the art of pulse diagnosis. This highly sophisticated system provides abundant information about the entire body, and it can easily take an entire lifetime to become truly proficient in this ancient diagnostic method. In an ideal situation, the pulse is taken in the morning while the person is still calm and rested. In actuality, however, the procedure usually takes place in the clinic during the initial interview. It is important to let patients who have just arrived rest for a while to allow the pulses to settle down. Otherwise, it would be easy to mistake a rapid pulse for a heat condition when it is actually due to the person's hurrying to make the appointment.

Although the pulse can be felt in a number of locations, the primary location is at the radial artery in the wrist. Each wrist has three positions that correspond to different organs. The left wrist corresponds to the heart, liver, and kidney yin. The right wrist gives information about the lungs, spleen, and kidney yang. These six positions are also felt at three different depths: deep, middle, and superficial. In addition to the information that can be gleaned from these 18 locations, the experienced practitioner can identify 28 different types of pulses. It's not hard to understand why it takes a lifetime of practice to become truly proficient at pulse-taking.

A normal pulse is strongest at the middle depth. In patterns of deficiency, the pulse is only palpable at the deepest levels. A person fighting off a cold will have a strong pulse at the superficial level due to the defensive qi rushing to the surface of the body. This "floating" pulse is fairly easy for a beginner to identify, and it can be very useful clinically. Many times, this pulse appears a couple of days before a person experiences any cold symptoms, making it possible to practice early intervention. Since a rapid pulse is a sign of heat and a slow pulse is a sign of cold, a floating, rapid pulse occurs if the condition is a case of wind heat. In this case, the pulse is also strong, since wind heat is an excess condition. A weak pulse, on the other hand, indicates a deficient condition. For example, a person with kidney yang deficiency has a deep, weak pulse, especially in the area on the right wrist that corresponds to kidney yang.

Since learning the pulses requires hands-on experience, a detailed description is beyond the scope of this book. In a clinical setting, however, students are trained to discern the following types of pulses: floating, sinking, slow, fast, empty, full, wiry, slippery, flooding, hollow, leather, soggy, hidden, confined, moderate, choppy, knotted, intermittent, hurried, spinning bean, tight, sick, scattered, small, minute, short, long, and frail. Each one of these pulses is associated with a variety of imbalances, and an experienced practitioner can learn an enormous amount of information from the pulse alone. In clinical practice, however, the physician always combines the pulse information with the whole picture derived from looking, listening, smelling, and asking. Through this process, traditional Chinese practitioners are able to accurately diagnose the patterns of imbalance in their patients without the help of laboratory tests or expensive diagnostic equipment.

TREATMENTS IN TRADITIONAL CHINESE MEDICINE

Once practitioners of traditional Chinese medicine make a diagnosis, they have the following options available to treat their patients: acupuncture, herbal medicine, moxibustion, cupping, exercise therapy, massage techniques, and dietary therapy. The most common therapeutic modalities are acupuncture and herbal medicine, which have such a wide range of applications, they are appropriate for most conditions. Moxibustion (the application of heat to acupuncture points or injured areas) is also widely used, while cupping (the application of suction cups to remove stagnation from an area) is often employed as an adjunct therapy for pain and stagnation. A traditional massage technique known as tui na has a profound effect on the musculoskeletal system. Finally, dietary therapy is an important aspect of all healing systems, and Chinese medicine is no exception. Foods are grouped according to the organ systems they affect and whether they are hot or cold, damp or dry, yin or yang. Practitioners often advise patients about which foods to eat and which to avoid for their particular imbalance.

ACUPUNCTURE

The practice of acupuncture is based on the flow of qi, or vital energy, through pathways in the body known as channels, or meridians. Twelve regular meridians correspond to each of the six yin and six yang organs—the spleen meridian to the spleen organ, the large intestine meridian to the large intestine organ, and so on. Eight extra meridians are also used in acupuncture therapy.

Disharmony in an organ often shows up in its corresponding meridian: A person experiencing a heart attack may also have a sensation of pain and numbness that travels down the arm into the little finger, closely following the path of the heart meridian. Practitioners palpate a diagnostic point on the corresponding meridian to assess the health of its related organ. In other cases, the meridians themselves are treated. A practitioner might treat a sore shoulder by increasing the flow of qi and blood through the large intestine, lung, and triple burner meridians. The organs related to these meridians may be completely healthy; these meridians are selected because they pass through the injured shoulder area.

WORLD HEALTH ORGANIZATION ENDORSES ACUPUNCTURE

The World Health Organization (WHO) is an international association of 190 countries with headquarters in Geneva, Switzerland. Traditional medicine is one of its many interests, since the organization recognizes that much of the world depends upon indigenous medicine. For over two decades, WHO has sponsored research into this field and has attempted to determine which traditional medical procedures are effective and which are not. The use of acupuncture has been supported by WHO since the 1970s.

Although they flow deep within the body, each meridian has specific points that can be accessed from the surface of the body. There are 361 such acupuncture points on the meridians, as well as numerous "extraordinary" points that may or may not be located on a regular channel. In addition, a full set of points on the ears represent all the organs in the body and can be used to treat a wide variety of medical conditions. Use of these points is known as auriculotherapy. Acupuncture points can be stimulated by means of pressure, heat, or needling. Each point has a specific set of functions. Some of these functions have local effects, while some are systemic. For example, the stomach meridian consists of 45 points, stretching from the head to the toes. A point just below the knee known as Dubi, or Stomach 35, is used almost exclusively for knee pain (a local effect), while the point just three inches below it, known as Zusanli (Stomach 36), has a systemic function. One of the most important points in acupuncture, Zusanli is used to treat stomach pain, vomiting, indigestion, diarrhea, constipation, dizziness, fatigue, and low immunity. Needling it often relieves stomach pain immediately. Modern research has confirmed that applying moxa or needles to this point actually raises the white blood cell count (white blood cells fight disease-causing organisms that invade the body).

Acupuncture has been practiced since ancient times with needles made from stone, wood, ivory, or bone. Modern practitioners use surgical-quality stainless steel needles with a handle wound with wire for a better grip. Some needles are plated with silver, gold, or copper to achieve special effects from the treatment, such as tonification or sedation, but the majority of needles are pure steel. In the past, needles were placed in an autoclave, a device used to sterilize dental and surgical tools, after each use. However, with the increase in prevalence of hepatitis and AIDS/HIV, most practitioners in the West now use presterilized disposable needles to ensure absolute safety. The needles are used only once and then discarded as medical waste, which gives peace of mind to the patients, practitioners, and insurance companies.

THE HISTORY OF ACUPUNCTURE

In China, the first ideas about medicine were gathered together at about the same time as the theory of yin and yang began to develop, during what is known as the Clan Period. This era began 100,000 years ago in the prehistoric period of Chinese civilization and is divided into two halves, known as the Old Stone Age and the New Stone Age. In these earliest times, medical knowledge was limited to basic skills such as dietary supplements, lancing and scraping infections, massage, herbal lore, and simple bone setting. Chinese scholars believe that it was in the New Stone Age, approximately 8000 to 2000 BC, that the science of acupuncture actually began. During this time, ongoing improvements in stone shaping techniques made it possible to manufacture the precise tools required. The legendary Yellow Emperor, Huang Di, (2690–2590 BC), is often credited with the creation of the first acupuncture needles and with developing techniques to use them. Renowned as a great benefactor of the people, he reportedly wrote *The Yellow Emperor's Classic of Internal Medicine*.

During this period, acupuncture needles were not the sharp, delicate tools we know today. In fact, the needles were made from stone. Known as "Bian Shyr," the needles of the time came in a number of different shapes and sizes. Some even looked remarkably like arrowheads.

Typically, the stones were used to lance an infection, to scrape an abscessed wound, or even to assist in bloodletting procedures. Five hundred years later, a technique known as moxibustion was introduced to work together with or independently from acupuncture.

Later discoveries from the Shang Dynasty (1776–1122 BC) demonstrated that thoughtful acupuncturists had inscribed bones and tortoise shells with symbols representing their medical knowledge. At roughly the same time, methods for casting bronze were developed, and needles made of this alloy began to appear. Still later, between what is known as the Warring States Period (465–221 BC) and the Western Han Dynasty (206 BC–AD 24), iron needles were created. These successfully displaced stone as the instrument of choice.

One hundred years later, around AD 100, needles of gold and silver were constructed. At least nine different shapes of needles were made, each for different purposes. Some needles, those that were sharp and thin, were used specifically for puncturing. Others, blunt and thick instruments, were used for massage. By this time, the ideas of yin and yang, the Five Element Theory, moxibustion, and the concepts of pulse, blood, chi, shen, and channels were firmly incorporated into the medical knowledge of the time.

Research with electrical conductivity has confirmed the real existence of acupuncture points, and double-blind studies have shown acupuncture is safe and effective in treating a wide range of diseases. Acupuncture is especially well known for its treatment of pain; it is so effective for pain relief, it is even used as a substitute for anesthesia in some surgical procedures in Chinese hospitals!

THE PRINCIPLE OF ACUPUNCTURE

Acupuncture treatment works on the principle that health is characterized by a smooth flow of qi and blood through the meridians and organs. When qi and blood become stagnant, pain occurs. If too much qi and blood are in a certain area, a syndrome of heat and excess can occur; too little qi and blood in an area results in a deficiency. During acupuncture treatment, the body undergoes normalization. Areas with too much qi and blood transfer these vital substances to areas that are deficient. The result is a process in which the body's innate wisdom brings about a self-regulatory effect. For example, the same acupuncture point can be used to treat either high or low blood pressure; similarly, another point is needled to treat both a rapid or slow heartbeat. This is one of the reasons acupuncture rarely causes side effects. It doesn't force the body to do anything; it only helps it to perform its normal functions.

THE TECHNIQUE

Many people are surprised to learn that acupuncture is relatively painless. Unlike hypodermic needles, which are hollow and much larger, acupuncture needles can be as fine as a human hair. Many times, a patient is not even aware a needle has been inserted, especially when it is placed in areas with relatively few sensory nerves, such as the back. In a typical acupuncture treatment, the patient lies down, and the practitioner inserts needles in points that have the desired effect on the body. The patient senses heaviness, movement, or an "electrical" impulse that signals the "arrival of qi." After a few minutes, the patient typically feels a sense of calmness and well-being; many people fall asleep.

After a period of 20 minutes to an hour, the practitioner removes the needles and advises the patient to avoid strenuous activity for a few hours to let the treatment settle in. Depending on the individual and the condition, one treatment might be sufficient, or the patient may need to return a number of times. Results can range from mild improvement to seemingly miraculous recovery. In almost all cases, however, the patient feels calmer and more peaceful after receiving acupuncture. Those who think acupuncture's success is merely a placebo effect or the patient's imagination should consider that acupuncture is exceptionally effective in animals. An increasing number of veterinarians specialize in acupuncture, and their results are quite dramatic.

In certain situations, acupuncture is inappropriate. It should not be performed if the patient is extremely hungry or full, intoxicated, or extremely fatigued. In these cases, the treatment may not be as effective or the person might experience dizziness or exhaustion. People with bleeding disorders such as hemophilia should also avoid acupuncture therapy, although careful application of acupressure or moxibustion is safe. A number of points should not be used during pregnancy due to their tendency to induce labor. Acupuncture is generally not used in children younger than 6 years of age.

ACUPRESSURE

Sometimes acupoints are stimulated using techniques other than acupuncture needles. Hands, for instance, have been used as healing tools since the beginning of time. Acupressure uses the fingers or palms rather than needles to apply pressure to acupoints. Entire channels can also be massaged in the hope of freeing the blocked energy within, promoting the flow of qi, and restoring good health. There are many systems of therapeutic massage, including Shiatsu, Jin Shin Do, and Tibetan massage.

Different oils are often used with massage techniques, and their proper use is associated with the seasons. Olive and sesame oils are used in winter while sandalwood oil can be used in summer. Some customs avoid massage altogether during the summer months.

HERBAL MEDICINE

Herbal medicine is as old as humanity itself. Early human beings were hunter-gatherers whose survival depended on their knowledge of their environment. Direct experience taught them which plants were toxic, which ones imparted strength and sustained life, and which had special healing qualities. These early discoveries were passed along until thousands of years and millions of human trials brought about the evolution of an incredibly sophisticated system of diagnosis and herbal medicine.

Thousands of medicinal substances are used in China today. Indeed, more than a million tons of herbs are used each year in China. Thirty herbs, mostly tonics, account for more than 50 percent of this figure, with licorice topping the list at 86,000 tons. This information may seem astonishing to the minds of Westerners, who see herbal medicine as a new development in healing. From a practical perspective, however, a fairly complete pharmacy stocks about 450 different individual herbs. From this collection of herbs, a clinical herbalist employs more than 250 standard formulas, each of which can be modified to fit a patient's individual pattern of disharmony.

The herbalist or practitioner combines herbs based on the diagnosis, using a traditional herbal formula as a foundation and adding other herbs specific to the individual's complaint and constitution. As the person's health improves, the nature of the imbalance changes, so the herb formula must also change. Some herbs are deleted when they are no longer needed, while others more appropriate to the changing condition are added.

CLASSIFICATION OF HERBAL MEDICINE

Herbs are classified according to whether they have a warming or cooling effect on the body. Their taste also has significance. Generally, sweet herbs tonify qi, sour herbs are astringent, bitter herbs dry damp and clear heat, acrid herbs disperse cold and stagnation, and salty herbs have a softening, purging effect. Both individual herbs and herbal formulas are organized into categories, based on diagnostic patterns. For example, if a person has deficient kidney yang, the practitioner selects herbs from the category of "herbs that tonify yang." The therapeutic categories of herbs follow:

Herbs that Release the Exterior: When the body's protective qi is repelling a pathogenic influence, the struggle occurs in the exterior layers of the body. Herbs in this category have an outward dispersing action, preventing the disease from penetrating to the interior of the body. Warm herbs of this type expel wind cold by inducing perspiration and warming the body; cool, acrid herbs are chosen to repel wind heat.

Herbs that Clear Heat: This category of cooling herbs clears all kinds of internal heat—excess heat, heat from deficiency, heat in the blood, heat with toxicity, and damp heat.

Downward Draining Herbs: These herbs treat differing degrees of constipation and are used as cathartics, purgatives, and mild lubricating laxatives.

Herbs that Drain Dampness: This category contains herbs that remove dampness in the form of edema or urinary disorders.

Herbs that Dispel Wind Dampness: Used mostly for arthritis and skin conditions, these herbs increase circulation and reduce swelling and inflammation.

Herbs that Transform Phlegm and Stop Coughing: Some of these herbs relax the cough reflex, others clear phlegm. For heat phlegm, cooling moistening expectorants are chosen; warming drying expectorants are used to treat cold phlegm.

Aromatic Herbs that Transform Dampness: If dampness overwhelms the digestive organs, these herbs penetrate the dampness with their aroma and revive the spleen.

Herbs that Relieve Food Stagnation: When food is stuck in the stomach, this category of herbs is chosen in order to move the stagnation.

Herbs that Regulate Qi: These herbs remove stagnation from the digestive system and move qi that is stuck in the liver.

Herbs that Regulate Blood: Herbs in this category are divided into those that stop bleeding and those that increase circulation and remove stagnation.

Herbs that Warm the Interior: Warming the metabolism at a deep level, these herbs dispel cold conditions and revive the digestive fire—the metabolic energy required to digest food. When it is low (as in spleen yang deficiency), digestion is weak and the person craves warm foods and liquids.

Tonifying Herbs: Divided into herbs that tonify yin, yang, qi, or blood, this is the superior category of medicines. These herbs can prevent disease rather than simply treat disease that has already appeared. Nourishing and strengthening, they can be used long-term to correct deficiencies of the vital substances (qi, blood, body fluids, essence).

Astringent Herbs: These herbs dry excessive secretions, such as diarrhea, excessive urination, or sweating.

Herbs that Calm the Spirit: These substances have a calming effect and are used for anxiety, insomnia, palpitations, and irritability.

Herbs that Open the Heart: Containing aromatic substances, usually resins, these herbs can revive a person's consciousness. Some are used for conditions such as angina.

Herbs that Clear Internal Wind and Tremors: These herbs treat muscle spasms, hypertension, and involuntary movements.

Herbs that Expel Parasites: These herbs can destroy or expel various parasites from the body.

Substances for External Application: These consist of herbs and minerals, many of them toxic if taken internally, that are applied topically for skin problems, bruises, spasms, and sprains.

Herbal formulas also are divided into the same diagnostic categories. The traditional formulas, or patent medicines, are an intricate combination of herbs chosen to address the various aspects of a disease pattern. The chief herb in the formula addresses the major complaint; the formula usually contains more of this particular herb than other herbs. The deputy herb assists the chief herb in its function, while the assistant herb reinforces the effects of the chief and deputy or performs a secondary function. The envoy directs the formula to a certain part of the body, or it harmonizes and detoxifies the other parts of the formula. For example, Ephedra Decoction is used for wind cold with wheezing, stiff neck from cold, and a lack of sweating. *Ephedra* is the chief herb, since it treats all of the main symptoms. Cinnamon twig is the deputy because it assists in promoting sweating and warming the body. Apricot seed acts as the assistant by focusing on the wheezing, while licorice is the envoy because it harmonizes the actions of the other herbs. Larger formulas may have multiple herbs that produce the different functions, depending on the desired action of the formula.

Herbs can be taken in the form of decoctions, pills, liquid extracts, powdered extracts, and syrups. Decoctions tend to be the strongest medicine, followed by concentrated liquid extracts, concentrated powdered extracts, and pills. All are effective, and the use of the different forms depends on the individual's personal choice. If you don't have the time to make a decoction or you don't like the taste, pills or capsules will be more effective, simply because you'll be more likely to take them. The concentrated liquid extracts tend to take effect quickly, so they are useful in cases where fast action is important, and the syrups are good for sore throats or as tonics. However, many of the more concentrated extracts are available only from a health care practitioner. In whatever form they are taken, though, accurately prescribed herbal formulas are exceptionally effective in restoring health and vitality.

MOXIBUSTION

Moxibustion, or moxa, is named after the Japanese word mokusa, meaning "burning herb." It was first recorded in medical texts during the Song Dynasty (AD 960), but it has most likely been in use much longer. It is an important therapy in traditional Chinese medicine; the ancient texts advise that moxa should be tried if acupuncture and herbs have failed to heal the disease. The heat from moxibustion is very penetrating, making it effective for impaired circulation, cold and damp conditions, and yang deficiency. When applied to acupuncture points specific for yang deficiency, the body absorbs the heat into its deepest levels, restoring the body's yang qi and "life-gate fire," the source of all heat and energy in the body. Moxa is prepared from mugwort (*Artemisia vulgaris*), which is a common perennial herb. The aromatic leaves are dried and repeatedly sifted until they are fluffy.

There are two techniques used to apply moxibustion: indirect moxa and direct moxa. In indirect moxa, the "moxa wool" is rolled into a cigar shape and wrapped in paper. The stick is then lighted and held about an inch away from the desired area—an acupuncture point or other area of the body chosen by the practitioner. Indirect moxa can be used on acupuncture points to achieve a systemic, or bodywide, effect or it can be used directly at the site of a problem. For example, indirect moxa might be applied to a swollen, stiff area such as an arthritic joint. It is also appropriate to apply indirect heat to specific acupuncture points, such as Zusanli (Stomach 36) or Mingmen (Du 4), to create a systemic effect. The heat taken into these points raises the body's metabolism and immunity, so moxibustion at these points can also be used in preventive health care. One ancient text declares that "one who applies moxa daily to Zusanli (Stomach 36) will be free of the one hundred diseases." Applying moxa to Stomach 36 has an energizing effect on the body, especially in regard to immune and digestive functions. Some indications for its use in Chinese medicine are to treat general weakness, anemia, indigestion, nausea, chronic fatigue, shock, allergies, and asthma.

Another type of indirect moxa involves rolling the moxa, placing it on the end of an acupuncture needle while the needle is in the body, and igniting it. The heat from the moxa travels down the handle and into the needle. The needle transfers the heat specifically to the desired point on the body.

In direct moxibustion, a small amount of herb is rolled into a cone and burned on the skin. This can cause a burn, so this technique is rarely performed in Western acupuncture clinics. In most cases when moxa is applied directly to the skin, some ointment is placed on the point. In other techniques, the moxa is burned on top of a slice of ginger, garlic, or aconite; this prevents a burn and adds the therapeutic effects of those herbs to the treatment.

In all cases, moxibustion can be a very pleasant sensation, especially when the warmth spreads through areas that have pain and swelling due to cold. Indirect moxa is also easy to learn to do at home. Practitioners often show a patient the appropriate point for their condition, and the person can take a moxa stick home to perform daily treatments. Such treatment can be very empowering, since the patient then takes responsibility for his own healing.

CUPPING

Cupping is a therapy in which a special cup or jar is attached to the skin by means of suction. The suction is created by heating the air inside the cup to create a vacuum, then quickly pressing the mouth of the cup to the desired area. There are also modern cups that can be applied with a suction device. Interestingly, cultures all over the world are known to use this technique, making it virtually a universal practice. In ancient times, it was done with bamboo cups or animal horns, and it was often employed to treat external conditions of the skin and muscles such as sprains and strains and drawing out pus. It is especially effective for musculoskeletal pain, often relieving the pain after a single application. The force of the suction draws stagnant blood to the surface of the body, sometimes leaving a round bruise in the shape of the cup. Since pain is caused by the stagnation of qi and blood, the goal of this therapy is to remove the stagnation, increase circulation, and allow healing to take place.

Cupping should not be used when the patient has broken skin, skin ulcers, edema, high fever, bleeding disorders, varicose veins, or convulsions. It should also not be performed on the abdomen or low back of a woman who is pregnant. Care needs to be taken to avoid burning the patient with a hot cup; using the cups with the suction device eliminates this potential problem.

EXERCISE

The practice of qi gong is exceptionally common in China. On any given morning, parks all over the country are filled with people of all ages practicing the graceful movements of qi gong. While most people perform these exercises for their own benefit, a practitioner can impart healing energy to a patient's body through medical qi gong methods.

QI GONG

Qi gong (pronounced chee guhng) has been practiced in China in its various forms for thousands of years. It consists of exercises involving specific breathing practices and/or movements, with the goal of enhancing and balancing qi. The central principle involves meditating on a vital energy center known as the Dantian (pronounced dahn tyehn). Located about three inches below the navel, it is considered the root of qi in the body. By focusing on this area while moving the body, a person is able to build up a storehouse of qi and direct it to areas that need it.

Qi gong has a wide variety of forms, ranging from quiet meditative exercises that bring about a sense of peace and well-being to techniques that send powerful waves of energy flowing through the body. In its medical form, qi gong is used to build immunity, treat disease, improve strength, clarify the mind, and enable a person to tap into underlying reserves of energy. The ancient Chinese physician Hua Tuo is quoted as saying "a running stream never goes bad," meaning that qi and blood will not become stagnant if proper exercise keeps them circulating. He developed a set of exercises known as "imitation of five animals boxing," which was an early form of qi gong. He and his followers were able to remain healthy into old age by practicing these exercises regularly.

As Chinese medicine grew more sophisticated over time, the practice of qi gong also became more focused on curing specific diseases. By the 1800s, it was used clinically for ailments such as indigestion, toothache, eye problems, headache, abdominal pain, and chronic degenerative diseases in general.

The practitioner of qi gong trains in order to master three groups of exercises: those that regulate the body, those that regulate the heart and mind, and those that regulate breathing. The purpose of these exercises is for the practitioner to learn to release muscular tension, strengthen the muscles and tendons, and circulate qi and blood to the various organs and regions of the body. Different positions are assumed, depending on the desired result, but in all cases a profound relaxation allows the muscles and organs to rest and rejuvenate. Meditating on the Dantian also allows the practitioner of qi gong to become free of distracting thoughts, bringing about a state of inner peace and heightened awareness. In medical qi gong, it is possible to direct the healing energy to specific organs and meridians. The patient can do this, and it is also possible for the physician to direct healing qi into the patient's body through his or her hands. When qi gong is combined with acupuncture treatment, the therapeutic results can be truly remarkable.

Much research into the physiologic effects of qi gong has been conducted in modern China. Studies have shown a drastic alteration of brain wave patterns and a radical decrease in adrenaline. Heart rate slows, blood pressure decreases, cholesterol levels can drop, and the immune system is strengthened by increased production of blood cells. Physicists studying the effects of qi gong at research institutes have actually discovered quantifiable changes during the practice of qi gong, such as the body's production of low levels of energy in the form of infrared energy, visible light, static electricity, and even ultraviolet and microwave radiation. Much more research remains to be done in this fascinating field, but one finding is certain: Qi gong is a powerful therapeutic modality capable of promoting wellness and healing disease. It stands well on its own and is also an effective adjunct to other traditional therapies.

THERAPEUTIC MASSAGE (TUI NA)

No healing modality could possibly be older than massage, since it is such a basic human instinct to rub a painful area. The Chinese have developed a sophisticated system of massage over a period of thousands of years that is used for numerous conditions. Going far beyond the expected applications for musculoskeletal pain, this massage technique is taught in Chinese medical schools, and specialists in the art are able to treat a wide range of diseases effectively. By working with the meridian system, practitioners are able to treat internal conditions such as hypertension, peptic ulcer, insomnia, nausea, arthritis, and constipation.

Pediatric massage is a field of specialty practiced in Chinese hospitals. It is especially effective on children younger than 5 years of age, and the younger the child, the more effective the treatment tends to be. The caress of a loving parent is the first sensation a baby experiences after birth, and recent research in the West has shown that infants who are routinely touched tend to be healthier and gain more weight. Some of the conditions treated by pediatric tui na, or massage, are diarrhea, vomiting, poor appetite, common cold, fever, bed-wetting, and crying at night. As in adult therapeutic massage, pediatric massage involves a variety of manipulations, such as pushing, spreading, kneading, pinching, and pressing. The manipulations are chosen according to the level of stimulation desired and the nature of the area massaged.

The results of Chinese therapeutic massage can often be quite dramatic, bringing about an immediate sense of healing. It is especially effective when used with other modalities, such as herbal medicine. For example, in an injury, herbs are taken internally to reduce the inflammation, swelling, and pain. In addition, a topical herb formula is combined with oil and massaged into the injured area to increase circulation and healing to the area, augmenting the systemic effect of the internal formula. This sort of three-pronged approach ensures a much faster recovery time, and it is one of the reasons that tui na practitioners are held in such high regard in China.

DIETARY THERAPY

Chinese dietary therapy is an integral part of any complete treatment plan. The earliest written record is Sun Simiao's **Prescriptions Worth a Thousand Gold**, published in AD 652, in which he discusses the treatment of a variety of diseases through diet. For example, his treatment for goiter included the use of seaweed and the thyroid glands from farm animals. This early iodine and hormone replacement therapy predates Western discoveries by hundreds of years. Similarly, in AD 752, Wang Shou published *A Collection of Diseases*, in which he describes his treatment for diabetes. He recommended the use of pork pancreas as a treatment, predating the discovery of insulin by 1,000 years. In the absence of laboratory tests, his method of checking for sugar in the urine was ingenious: The patient was instructed to urinate on a flat brick to see if ants would show up to collect the sugar!

In the traditional system of dietary cures, foods have been organized into categories based on their innate temperature, energetics (the direction in which they move qi and how they affect qi and blood flow), and the organs they affect. For example, a person who has a wind cold condition with excessive clear mucus might be told to consume hot soup made from onions and mustard greens. The onions are warming, expel cold, and sedate excess yin. The mustard greens have similar properties, and they also help expel mucus and relieve chest congestion. Flavoring the soup with ginger and black pepper enhances the warming, expectorant action. With such a lunch, one can imagine that the person's herb formula would be much more effective. On the other hand, if the same patient decided to have salad for lunch with a cold glass of milk, the cold and damp nature of this meal would make the wind cold condition much worse. Any herbal therapy administered at this point would be much less effective, since the therapy first needs to overcome the negative effect of the food before dealing with the acute ailment. For this reason, a patient is always advised about which foods could exacerbate the imbalance and which will help restore balance.

In general, grains and beans are considered to bring stability to the body. They build blood and qi, and they establish rhythm and stability. Vegetables, which are best if eaten in season, bring vitality. Leafy greens have an affinity for the upper body, while root vegetables give strength to the middle and lower body. Fruits build fluids and purge toxins, and they tend to be cooling by nature. They should be eaten alone, or they can cause indigestion. Meats possess the full range of temperatures, and they are a simple source of blood. But they are meant to be consumed in small quantities; their overconsumption in Western countries has caused an epidemic of heart disease. Finally, dairy products are a good source of fats, but they should also be eaten in moderation. Over-consumption can result in excess dampness or mucus. A healthy diet should consist mainly of a wide variety of organically grown whole grains, beans, and vegetables; fruits and animal protein should be eaten in smaller amounts.

A TYPICAL TREATMENT PLAN

A practitioner of traditional Chinese medicine may specialize in acupuncture only or herbal medicine only; some practice both. On its own, each therapy system can treat a wide range of diseases. However, most practitioners agree that a highly effective treatment consists of a combination of the two. A typical treatment plan might consist of an acupuncture treatment once a week with herbs taken between treatments. This combination of acupuncture and herbal therapy is applied often in the West, where most people must pay out of their own pockets for acupuncture treatments. In China's socialized medical system, a person might receive free acupuncture daily for two weeks as a course of treatment, take a break for a few days, and then undergo another course of treatment. But in the West, unless a patient's insurance policy covers alterna-tive medical practices, this sort of treatment plan is simply too expensive for most people. Using herbal therapy between acupuncture treatments provides continuous treatment at a lower cost to the patient.

There is no typical duration of treatment in traditional Chinese medicine, since each case is treated individually. A person with an acute, but simple, con-dition might feel completely free of illness and pain after just one acupuncture treatment, while another person with a chronic disorder might require weekly acupuncture and daily herbal medicine for a few months before the condi-tion is rectified. In all cases, however, the practitioner chooses the treatment modality he or she believes will be most effective in view of the practitioner's experience and the individual receiving treatment.

While all the treatment methods described here are part of an ancient tradi-tion, Chinese medicine continues to evolve. New treatment modalities have been tested and introduced, such as electroacupuncture (in which a mild elec-trical current is applied to the needles to provide a stronger and more contin-uous stimulation—a useful technique when stronger stimulation is desired, as in cases of paralysis), magnetic therapy, laser acupuncture (in which the points are stimulated with a special laser, a technique favored by people afraid of needles), and various types of healing radiation. With the wealth of knowledge from the past joining the ingenuity of the future, traditional Chinese medicine possesses a powerful set of tools for the treatment of disharmony and disease in all its forms.

TREATMENT OF COMMON AILMENTS

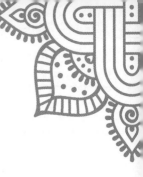

This chapter describes some common ailments that can be treated successfully with traditional Chinese medicine. Each disorder is explained in the context of possible Chinese diagnoses, and a typical treatment plan is described. Treatment might include a combination of acupuncture, herbal medicine, moxibustion, qi gong, and massage therapy, depending on the ailment. Treatment also depends on the style and training of the practitioner: Some specialize in acupuncture alone, while others rely mostly on herbs or other modalities. Still, the most common treatment plan is a combination of acupuncture and herbal medicine, and this is reflected in the sample treatment plans in this chapter. A practitioner may create an herbal formula specifically for your condition or prescribe a Chinese patent medicine.

ALLERGIES

Allergies occur when the body's immune system misidentifies a normally harmless substance as a threat. Common allergens are foods, pollen, animal dander, mold, insect venom, drugs, and dust mites. An inflammatory reaction takes place in an attempt to eject this substance, resulting in a variety of symptoms. A traditional Chinese medical treatment for pollen allergies, or hay fever, follows.

It is very important to remember that the purpose of this section on ailments and the following section is to give an idea of how a practitioner of Chinese medicine views and treats common ailments. *The information is not meant to replace qualified medical care, nor is it in any way intended to be a complete discussion of the given ailments.* After consulting this book, seek the help of a qualified health care practitioner for an accurate diagnosis and treatment plan.

Several Chinese patterns of disharmony may be involved in cases of allergies. In all cases, however, wind is part of the diagnosis, usually combining with another pathogenic influence in wind dampness, wind cold, or wind heat. Typical of patterns involving wind, allergy symptoms often occur without warning. In seasonal allergies, such as hay fever, the most common diagnosis is wind and dampness. This combination produces a sudden onset of symptoms: sneezing, itching eyes and throat, and a heavy sensation in the head with copious mucus. The treatment strategy is to repel the wind with herbs that are dispersing in nature, such as Japanese catnip (*Schizonepeta tenuifolia*, jing jie) and *Siler divaricata* (fang feng). Herbs that drain dampness are also employed in order to clear the nasal passages and sinuses; the major herbs for this purpose are *Angelica dahurica* (bai zhi), magnolia flower buds (xin yi hua), and *Xanthium sibiricum* (cang er zi). This combination is known as Xanthium Decoction. An appropriate patent medicine is Bi Yan Pian.

Typically, an underlying weakness, often a deficiency of lung and spleen qi, makes persons with allergies susceptible to allergic reactions. Lung qi is responsible for the proper function of the entire respiratory tract, including the nasal passages. Spleen qi controls the transport of fluids; when spleen qi is impaired, weakening digestive function, it can lead to an overproduction of mucus, which tends to collect in the lungs. This weakness of qi is treated with tonifying herbs that bolster lung and spleen function, such as *Codonopsis* (dang shen), *Atractylodes* (bai zhu), *Poria* (fu ling), and prepared licorice (zhi gan cao). An appropriate patent medicine for this type of deficiency is Six Gentlemen Teapills. This formula also contains *Pinellia* (ban xia) and aged citrus peel (chen pi), which enhance the base formula's ability to clear mucus and dry dampness. A traditional Chinese medicine practitioner may customize the formula to meet a patient's individual needs. For example, *Chrysanthemum* flowers (jua hua) and *Cassia* seeds (jue ming zi) can be added to soothe itchy eyes, and jujube dates (da zao) can be included to enhance the overall antiallergic action of the formula.

Diet plays an important part in controlling seasonal allergies. Sweets, dairy products, and cold foods all tend to increase mucus buildup, putting ice cream and yogurt at the top of the list of foods to avoid during allergy season. When excessive mucus accumulates in the system, allergens stimulate a much stronger allergic reaction. Soups, salads (in warm weather), vegetables, and boiled grains are all easy for the body to digest. When digestion is efficient, there is less of a tendency for mucus to build up.

Treatment plans for allergies vary greatly, and the possible results range from temporary relief to complete remission. Acupuncture frequently relieves allergy symptoms immediately. Manipulation of points around the nose, such as Yintang, Bitong, and Large Intestine 20, usually relieves the nasal congestion and sneezing as soon as the needles are inserted.

Recently, a similar but more sophisticated system of allergy-elimination acupuncture has been developed in which the acupuncture is performed while the person is exposed to the allergen. Developed by Dr. Devi Nambudripad, this technique is called Nambudripad's Allergy Elimination Technique (NAET). The patient undergoes allergy testing to identify the allergen. Then acupressure and acupuncture techniques are used to clear the allergen while the patient is exposed to it. This treatment reprograms the body to accept the allergen without producing an allergic reaction. The effects are long-term, and the allergy is virtually eliminated.

ARTHRITIS

Arthritis is a degenerative inflammatory disease that attacks the joints in particular, causing symptoms of stiffness, swelling, pain, and loss of the normal range of motion. It is especially common in elderly people, although rheumatoid arthritis can occur in young people as well. In traditional Chinese patterns of disharmony, the various types of arthritis fall typically under the category of "painful obstruction syndrome." Acute painful obstruction can be due to wind, cold, dampness, or heat, although it is usually a combination of wind, dampness, and cold. In an acute attack of wind, cold, and dampness, symptoms include joint pain that gets worse with cold and is relieved with warmth, a feeling of heaviness or numbness in the limbs, limited mobility of the affected area, and, possibly, a slow pulse. A more chronic arthritis condition is generally associated with an underlying deficiency of the vital substances involving the liver and kidneys, in view of their relationship to the tendons and bones.

The most common Western treatment for arthritis is non-steroidal anti-inflammatory drugs (NSAIDS). Although these drugs can relieve pain and decrease inflammation, they do nothing to cure the disease. Traditional Chinese treatments also reduce pain and inflammation, but they focus on eliminating the cause of the arthritis. Arthritis responds well to acupuncture. When combined with moxa, it can relieve pain and reduce inflammation immediately. Some acute cases require only a few treatments. Needles are typically placed into points surrounding the painful area, bringing circulation to the area and helping relieve the stagnation that causes pain and swelling. A more chronic, long-term arthritic condition can take months or even years to resolve. For this reason, it is essential to begin treating this disorder at an early stage.

Herbal therapy is especially important as part of the treatment of chronic cases. The treatment strategy varies, depending on whether the condition is due to heat or cold, or if there is a deficiency of any vital substances. Herbal remedies in chronic cases of cold and dampness need to nourish the underlying deficiency as well as expel the cold and dampness. The patent formula for this condition is Du Huo Ji Sheng Wan. The most effective formula is one custom-made for the patient's individual constitution and pattern of disharmony.

In any type of arthritis, it is important to get regular exercise to warm the body and get the qi and blood flowing. If the pattern involves cold and dampness, the diet should consist mostly of cooked foods with moderate amounts of anti-inflammatory spices such as cayenne and ginger. Although coffee is warming, it should be avoided due to its irritating nature.

COMMON COLD

The common cold has many forms in traditional Chinese medicine. The most common forms fall under the categories of wind cold and wind heat. As is the nature of exterior disorders involving wind, the pattern may change very quickly, necessitating a change in treatment strategy over the course of an illness. In all the forms a cold, as well as a cough or the flu, may take, prompt treatment brings the most effective results. The longer one waits to treat an infectious disease, the longer it takes to clear the pathogen.

Wind Cold: This pattern exhibits the following symptoms: fever, chills (these are worse than the fever), inability to get warm, nasal or sinus congestion with clear mucus, cough with clear mucus, stiff neck and shoulders, occipital headache (back of head), and a slower-than-normal pulse that is more easily felt at the surface. Diaphoretic (sweating) therapy is especially helpful in this condition, since it warms the body and pushes the pathogen out through the pores. In the very early stages of this pattern, an effective remedy is miso soup with the white part of spring onion (cong bai) and fresh ginger (sheng jiang). For more severe or advanced cases, there is a full range of therapies.

When the wind-cold symptoms include strong chills, inability to sweat, wheezing, and stiff neck, the classic and ancient remedy is Ephedra Decoction (Ma Huang Tang). The chief herb in this formula is *Ephedra* (ma huang), a powerful stimulant that opens the bronchial passages, warms the body, and stimulates sweating. Cinnamon twig (gui zhi) assists the *Ephedra* in warming the body and promoting a sweat, while apricot seeds (xing ren) help relieve the wheezing. Licorice (gan cao) acts as a harmonizing herb, modulating the harsh nature of the *Ephedra*, preventing too much sweating and toxicity. It also has anti-inflammatory and antitussive qualities, making it useful for sore throat and cough symptoms. *Ephedra* is never used by itself in Chinese herbal therapy; it is always part of a formula, often combined with licorice (as in Ephedra Decoction), which tones down its harsh nature. Since *Ephedra* can raise blood pressure, especially when used alone or with caffeine, it should not be used by people who have heart disease or hypertension. For symptoms of wind cold with headache and nasal congestion as the chief symptoms, the classic formula is Chuan Xiong Cha Tiao Wan, typically taken with green tea (cha), which moves the action of the formula to the head area. Green tea has been found recently to have strong antioxidant properties, scavenging the free radicals involved in aging and disease.

Wind Heat: When the pernicious influence of wind combines with heat, the fever is worse than the chills, and the pulse is faster than normal. The primary symptom is a swollen and sore throat with headache and irritability. If there is a cough, it is usually dry or nonproductive, with occasional expectoration of yellow mucus. Numerous formulas treat the many variations of this condition, but the most famous by far is Yin Qiao San. This highly effective treatment for wind heat symptoms, appearing in such conditions as influenza and tonsillitis as well as the common cold, is also available from a number of different manufacturers as the patent formula Yin Qiao Jie Du Pian.

In addition to Yin Qiao, a number of effective remedies are discussed in the section on patent medicines (next chapter). For example, Gan Mao Ling is almost always useful in cases of wind heat. If the fever is high, Zhong Gan Ling is preferred. If the sore throat is especially severe, it is recommended to add Chuan Xin Lian Antiphlogistic Tablets to the treatment.

When treating cold or flu symptoms due to wind heat, the results are always more dramatic if treatment begins early. It is important to get adequate rest, a vacation from sources of stress, and good nutrition in the form of soups and fresh juices. Sweets and stimulants (such as caffeinated beverages) cause a rapid progression in the severity of the illness since they tend to feed the pathogen. The same is true for tonifying herbs such as ginseng. People sometimes make the mistake of taking ginseng when they feel a cold coming on since they have heard that ginseng is good for the immune system. Using ginseng in this case is a serious error since ginseng will feed the pathogen causing the illness, making the person feel worse. A powerful tonic herb, ginseng acts to "lock down" the exterior of the body while releasing energy in the interior. If a pathogen is already inside the body, ginseng and other stimulating tonics lock it in while simultaneously feeding it. The proper treatment plan is to open the pores and push out the pathogen. Herb formulas that "release the exterior and repel wind," such as Yin Qiao, are used in these cases.

On the other hand, if no pathogen is in the body, ginseng strengthens the wei qi, the body's wall against invaders, while it simultaneously improves the person's vitality and resistance to disease. This distinction between building long-term immunity and fighting off an acute illness is an important contribution of traditional Chinese medicine. While tonic herbs can be taken long-term, it is important to discontinue their use during a cold or flu. Then, after the pathogen has been expelled from the body, tonic herbs can be taken again to build up strength and vitality over the long-term.

Acupuncture and moxibustion can provide some immediate relief from cold symptoms and help the body expel the pathogen much faster. Needles are typically inserted into points along the lung and large intestine meridians, which have demonstrated the ability to activate immune function. The most important acupuncture point in treating the common cold is Large Intestine 4 ("Adjoining Valleys"), which is located in the web between the thumb and index finger. This point is very effective for this condition, since it suppresses pain and relieves exterior conditions. Patients frequently experience quick relief when the point is needled or massaged. Typically, one or two acupuncture treatments and a week's course of herbal medicine are all that are required for colds. If the symptoms are recognized and treated early, it is possible to fight off a cold in a day or two with acupuncture treatment and herbs.

CONSTIPATION

If you notice a sudden change in your bathroom habits, have to strain to move your bowels, or feel uncomfortable even after you've attempted to have a bowel movement, you may be constipated, which happens when stools pass too slowly through your intestines. Constipation can have many causes, including not getting enough fluids, dietary fiber, or physical activity; not going to the bathroom when you feel the urge; use of certain drugs; and overuse of laxative. Constipation is also related to some serious health conditions such as depression, hyperthyroidism, and colon cancer.

A number of patterns of disharmony, both excess and deficiency, can cause constipation. The excess patterns are excess heat and qi stagnation. When exterior heat penetrates into the interior, it can affect the large intestine, with symptoms of high fever, thirst, and sweating. The pulse is full and rapid, and the tongue is red with a yellow coat. In this case, herbs are selected that have a cooling, purgative effect such as rhubarb root (da huang). A simple but effective formula for this condition is Xiao Cheng Qi Tang ("Less Drastic Purgative Decoction"). The patent formula, Peach Kernel Pills, is an effective remedy for less severe cases of constipation due to excess heat.

Constipation due to stagnant qi typically gets worse when the person is under stress. In this case, herbs are given that relax stuck qi and restore intestinal function. A good combination of patent medicines to take for this pattern is Xiao Yao Wan and Mu Xiang Shun Qi Wan. A deficiency of qi, blood, yin, or yang can also cause constipation. When qi is deficient, the person does not have the energy to move the bowels and often feels exhausted after trying. A person with this condition has a pale face and tongue and may break into a sweat while defecating. A good patent remedy for this condition is Shen Qi Da Bu Wan, which contains qi tonics such as *Astragalus* (huang qi) and *Codonopsis* (dang shen). *Cannabis* seeds (huo ma ren) are a good addition, since they are a nourishing, lubricating laxative. They are available in the form of hemp seed oil. If yang is also deficient, the person feels cold and may have low back pain. In this case, the formula should also contain *Cistanches* (rou cong rong); the patient should eat walnuts (hu tao ren), a lubricating yang tonic.

If yin deficiency is the underlying cause, the person has small, hard, dry stools, thirst, night sweats, and a red tongue with little or no coating. The patent medicine Rehmannia Teapills with the addition of some hemp seed oil is appropriate in this pattern.

Acute constipation is relatively easy to resolve with one or two acupuncture treatments and herbal laxatives. The most important acupuncture point for this condition is Stomach 25 ("Heaven's Axis"), located on either side of the navel. Depending on the severity of the constipation, herbal laxatives ranging in strengths from mild lubricants to strong purgatives can usually bring relief within a day. Chronic constipation is typically due to a deficiency in one of the vital substances, making tonifying herbs the treatment of choice. The herbs and acupuncture points are selected according to which vital substance needs to be nourished. Fully correcting the imbalance can take anywhere from a few days to a few months, with a weekly acupuncture treatment acting to keep qi flowing through the intestines.

COUGH

Traditional Chinese medicine is very effective in the treatment of coughs because of its differentiation of the various types. For example, a cough due to heat produces sticky phlegm that is difficult to expectorate; it is treated with cooling, moistening herbs and acupuncture points that clear heat from the lungs. On the other hand, a cough due to cold is accompanied by chills and copious mucus; it is treated with warming, drying herbs and the application of moxibustion. Without this differentiation, it is easy to see how an unfocused treatment might be ineffective or even cause the cough to get worse. Descriptions of a few of the more commonly diagnosed types of coughs follow.

Hot Phlegm Cough: In this syndrome, the accumulated phlegm becomes thick and sticky due to heat. The cough can have a loud, barking sound. The phlegm is quite difficult to expectorate and the heat gives it a darker color, ranging from yellow to brown or dark green. This type of cough requires aggressive treatment as the green indicates that the trapped mucus has become infected. Mucus in the lungs is an ideal breeding ground for bacteria, so it is important to clear the mucus as quickly as possible with herbs that moisten the lungs to dislodge the mucus and stimulate expectoration. A highly effective formula for this condition is Pinellia Expectorant Pills. This patent medicine is available under several names, including Qing Qi Hua Tan Wan or Pinellia Root Teapills, but they are all the same formula. To maximize the effect, it is best to take it along with Gan Mao Ling or Yin Qiao Jie Du Pian. As in all syndromes involving phlegm, diet is extremely important. It is best to avoid cold foods, dairy products, and sweets, as these all create mucus. Therapeutic foods include hot soups, cooked vegetables and whole grains, and small amounts of raw juices at room temperature to assist in moistening the lungs in order to promote expectoration.

Damp or Cold Phlegm Cough: This pattern is characterized by frequent coughing with expectoration of copious amounts of clear or sticky white phlegm that is typically more plentiful in the morning or after meals. There can also be nausea, a sensation of fullness in the chest or abdomen, poor appetite, fatigue, and a sensation of heaviness. The principle treatment in this syndrome is to clear the phlegm from the lungs and strengthen the digestion, since an underlying deficiency in spleen qi creates an inclination toward excessive mucus production. The classic formula for this condition is Er Chen Tang, or "Two Old Things Decoction," with the addition of herbs to repel the pathogen and warm the lungs. The patent version of Er Chen Tang is Er Chen Wan. If there are accompanying wind-cold symptoms of headache, stiff neck, and nasal congestion, the patent medicine Chuan Xiong Cha Tiao Wan can also be taken. Dietary therapy is similar to that for hot phlegm cough, except the avoidance of cold foods is very important. A person with this condition should consume lots of hot liquids, especially ginger tea, get plenty of rest, and stay warm. Hot soup made mostly from vegetables is a tasty treatment as well.

Wind Dryness Cough: This type of cough is typically contracted after exposure to a dry environment. Different from a chronic dry cough caused by a deficiency of lung yin (often from smoking), in this case the dryness of the air allows the dryness external pernicious influence to attack the lungs. The symptoms are a dry cough and a sore throat with a ticklish sensation, dry lips and mouth, and, possibly, a headache. The treatment principle is to repel the dryness pernicious influence, moisten the lungs, and stop the cough. A classic formula for this condition is Sang Xing Tang (pronounced sahng shing tahng), translated as "Mulberry Leaf and Apricot Seed Decoction." This formula doesn't come in a patent medicine, but an effective replacement is Chuan Bei Pi Pa Gao. The diet should consist of soups and plenty of liquids. When the condition is gone, it would be wise to begin taking American ginseng (xi yang shen) on a daily basis for a few weeks. This will strengthen the qi and yin of the lungs and make a future attack less likely.

Most acute coughs respond to the above treatments within a week, unless the person fails to improve their diet and get some rest. In that case, the cough can linger for weeks, often leading to a series of colds due to weakened immunity. Acupuncture therapy is very helpful in treating coughs due to any cause. Needling a point on the Conception Vessel meridian (an extra meridian) just above the sternum can quickly calm a cough and assist breathing. Moxa therapy is used typically in the cold, damp type of cough, since there is a need for warmth in that pattern.

DIARRHEA

The causes of diarrhea vary. In acute cases, a person can become dehydrated very quickly, so it is important to seek immediate medical attention if the condition persists. If an acute case of diarrhea occurs along with a common cold or stomach upset and it is accompanied by nausea, vomiting, and a lack of appetite, a reliable remedy is Huo Xiang Zheng Qi Wan.

If contaminated food or water is the cause, the diarrhea is often accompanied by a burning sensation and a strong smell. In these cases, a practitioner provides treatment to kill the pathogen (usually bacteria) with a formula such as Huang Lian Su Pian and restore normal digestive function with a formula such as Mu Xiang Shun Qi Wan. Most practitioners recommend a laboratory test to ensure the pathogens are eliminated.

In cases of chronic loose stools, the underlying pattern is usually spleen qi deficiency. Other symptoms might be fatigue, poor appetite, pale face and tongue, and gurgling sounds in the intestines. Shen Ling Bai Zhu Pian is an effective remedy in this pattern: The *Codonopsis* and *Atractylodes* herbs tonify the spleen, while its astringent herbs, such as lotus seeds, stop the diarrhea.

Acute diarrhea is fairly easy to treat with one or two acupuncture treatments and a few days of herbal therapy. Two points on the stomach meridian (25 and 37) are especially effective; relief comes soon after they are needled. If the diarrhea is chronic and due to qi or yang deficiency, moxibustion is very helpful when applied to these points. If the cause of discomfort is bacteria or parasites, herbal therapy as described above is the recommended treatment. The length of time needed to treat chronic cases varies; ultimately, the person's dietary habits are usually the decisive factor. Cases due to severe qi deficiency can take a few weeks to months to resolve. In all types of diarrhea, it is important to drink sufficient liquids to avoid dehydration. Hot peppermint tea or vegetable broth are good choices. Plain white rice is the best solid food to soothe the stomach and firm up the stools until the condition passes.

FATIGUE

Fatigue is a symptom of many different disorders, both psychological and physical. It is often difficult to discover its cause with modern Western diagnostic methods. Fortunately, diagnosing and treating this sort of generalized complaint is one of the strong points of Chinese medicine.

The first and most important step is to examine the person's lifestyle to eliminate any possible causes of fatigue, such as lack of sleep, poor diet, insufficient exercise, or overworking. Without correcting these problems, it is difficult or impossible to restore the patient's energy level. Once the proper lifestyle adjustments are made, treatment, particularly moxibustion and herbal therapy, are much more likely to be effective.

The most common diagnoses in cases of chronic fatigue are deficiency of qi, blood, or yang, and many cases are a combination of these syndromes. In cases of qi deficiency, there may be no physical abnormality, but the body lacks sufficient energy to perform various functions. In addition to fatigue, the patient has a weak pulse, pale tongue, bright pale face, and, possibly, shortness of breath and poor appetite, depending on the organs involved. Most qi ton-ics boost energy by improving the function of the lungs, spleen, and kidneys. Some appropriate patent remedies to rectify qi deficiency are Bu Zhong Yi Qi Wan, Nu Ke Ba Zhen Wan, Shen Qi Da Bu Wan, Extractum Astragali, and Ginseng Royal Jelly Vials. Typically, these herbal remedies are taken for a few months, since chronic deficiency syndromes take longer to rectify. Acupunc-ture therapy is administered to bring energy to deficient organs, and moxi-bustion is applied to important systemic points to bring new energy into the body. Acupuncture points are selected that tonify the vital substances, since a deficiency of one or more of them is usually the underlying cause of fatigue. The most important tonifying points are Stomach 36, Spleen 6, Kidney 3, Du 4, and Ren 4. When these points are activated with acupuncture and moxa, the entire body becomes energized. When combined with herbal therapy, a course of treatment typically takes place over a few weeks or months, depend-ing on the severity of the problem.

In cases of blood deficiency, there is insufficient blood to nourish the organs and tissues of the body. In mild cases, the blood count may be within the normal range, while more severe cases are diagnosed as anemia, which can oc-cur as a result of decreased bone marrow function, vitamin or iron deficiency, general malnutrition, blood loss from excessive menstrual flow, or an abnor-mal destruction of red blood cells. In traditional Chinese medicine, anemia is associated with a deficiency of vital substances in the heart, liver, spleen, and kidneys. Herbal therapy and moxibustion are frequently successful in normal-izing the blood count, no matter what the underlying pattern of disharmony is. Such therapy is closely monitored with regular blood tests, since anemia can have serious consequences if it persists. A typical course of treatment—a week-ly acupuncture and moxa session and daily use of tonifying herbs—might take a few months. Two of the important acupuncture points for anemia are Spleen 10 ("Sea of Blood") and Stomach 36 ("Leg Three Miles"). Spleen 10 is chosen for its regulatory effect on the blood, while Stomach 36 improves the assimila-tion of nutrients from food, aiding in the production of new blood cells.

A deficiency of both spleen qi and heart blood produces dizziness, poor ap-petite, and fatigue, with a pale face and tongue. The standard formula for this pattern is Kwei Be Wan. In addition, longan fruit can be eaten as is or boiled. It is sold in dried form, but in tropical climates it can be found fresh. It nour-ishes the heart blood, making it a good supplement to herbal therapy. If the underlying disharmony is liver and kidney yin deficiency, symptoms are fa-tigue, blurry vision, low back pain, sexual dysfunction, leg weakness, and night sweats. The treatment principle is to tonify liver and kidney yin with Rehm-annia Teapills. Another tasty fruit, *Lycium* berries (gou qi zi), can be added as a supplement for this pattern. The berries replenish the yin of the liver and kidneys, nourish the blood, and improve eyesight.

When anemia is the result of spleen and kidney yang deficiency, fatigue, a pale face and tongue, lack of libido, cold limbs, and loose stools can occur. Moxibustion is especially helpful in this pattern. Also, the person should avoid cold foods. In this case, a good patent remedy is Nu Ke Ba Zhen Wan, which tonifies both qi and blood. In addition, a decoction made of 10 grams dried ginger and 10 grams cinnamon bark tonifies the yang qi.

In all types of anemia, another patent medicine, Tang Kwei Gin, a pleasant-tasting liquid supplement, further builds the blood. The diet should be especially nutritious, with generous amounts of dark greens and legumes at most meals. Refined foods such as pastas, breads, and pastries should be avoided, since they are filling but provide very little nutrition.

HEADACHE

Headaches can occur in a variety of disease patterns in traditional Chinese medicine. Some headaches are associated with external pernicious influences, such as wind cold, wind heat, or wind damp. Others occur as a symptom of internal imbalances, such as liver fire, phlegm, blood stagnation, qi deficiency, or blood deficiency. It is especially important to have an accurate diagnosis when treating a headache, since the wrong treatment can actually make the condition worse.

When a headache is caused by an external pernicious influence, it can occur suddenly, often along with other symptoms of wind. When it is due to wind cold, the pain is typically in the back or the top of the head. Other symptoms could be an aversion to cold, tight and sore shoulders and neck, and nasal congestion. The classic formula for this pattern is Chuan Xiong Cha Tiao Wan taken along with green tea. When wind heat is the culprit, the headache can be quite severe. Other symptoms may be fever, sore throat, thirst, and a floating, rapid pulse. In this case, the appropriate formula is Yin Qiao Jie Du Pian or Gan Mao Ling. When the external pathogen is dampness, the pain is dull and the head feels heavy—as if it is wrapped in a wet blanket. There can also be fever or chills, nasal congestion, foggy thinking, and fatigue. An effective patent remedy for this type of headache is Huo Xiang Zheng Qi Wan, which is also appropriate for headaches due to internal dampness. In all the above types of acute, externally contracted headaches, the pain may be due, in part, to pressure in the sinuses. If any nasal or sinus congestion accompanies the headache, it is a good idea to take Bi Yan Pian also.

A common internal cause of headache is liver yang rising up to the head, which may occur when a person experiences anger or frustration, or it can be a result of long-term deficiency of liver yin. Symptoms are dizziness, irritability, and nausea; the headache is a throbbing pain on the sides of the head or behind the eyes. The classic formula for this condition is Tian Ma Gou Teng Yin, which is also quite effective in relieving tight neck and shoulders that can accompany the headache. It contains two herbs specific for headaches due to liver imbalances. In the condition known as liver fire, a condition of extreme heat, the symptoms are the same as for liver yang headaches, with the addition of red face and eyes, more severe anger, and a red tongue with a yellow coat. The standard formula for this pattern is Long Dan Xie Gan Wan, which purges heat from the liver. Symptoms of blood stagnation headaches are a sharp, fixed, stabbing pain in a specific location, a wiry, choppy pulse, and a purple tongue. Usually, previous traumatic injury caused the blood stagnation. Herbs are selected that move the blood and help to relieve pain, such as Yan Hu Suo Zhi Tong Pian.

A headache due to qi deficiency typically begins or gets worse after physical exertion, and it tends to feel better in the morning or after rest. A dull pain, it can be accompanied by fatigue and a poor appetite. The treatment principle in this case is to tonify qi. Some appropriate patent remedies are Bu Zhong Yi Qi Wan or Shen Qi Da Bu Wan.

If blood deficiency is the cause, the pain is dull but a little more severe than the pain of qi deficiency. A pale face and tongue, dizziness, blurry vision, and a small, thin pulse are typical symptoms. The pain begins or gets worse when the person is hungry or after the menstrual period. The classic formula, Nu Ke Ba Zhen Wan, tonifies qi and blood. Also, Tang Kwei Gin or Shou Wu Chih are effective blood tonics in a convenient, good-tasting liquid form.

In all types of headaches, acupuncture is a powerful tool, frequently relieving the pain within minutes. A point used for all types of headaches is Large Intestine 4 ("Adjoining Valleys"), since it relieves pain in general and is a specific point for conditions affecting the head. Other points are selected according to the location of the pain, such as the back of the head (Gallbladder 20), the temples (Taiyang), or the forehead (Stomach 8).

Following the treatment, it is important to incorporate some lifestyle and dietary modifications to eliminate the underlying cause of the headaches. For example, when the cause is liver heat, spicy and greasy foods should be avoided, and stress reduction should be a high priority. If the underlying pattern is qi or blood deficiency, the diet should be modified to incorporate more whole grains and beans, nuts, dark greens, and fresh, organic vegetables. Animal products tonify qi and blood, but they should be eaten in smaller quantities than the other foods. The protein, fats, and other nutrients they contain make them useful in rebuilding the body in cases of deficiency, but these same qualities make them factors in heart disease and cancer when eaten in excess.

INDIGESTION

Overeating or combining foods that are difficult to digest leads to acute indigestion or a condition known in Chinese medicine as food stagnation. Symptoms include a lack of appetite and an aversion to food, a full, bloated feeling in the stomach, nausea, vomiting, bad breath, and acid belching. The treatment principle is to move qi in the stomach, thereby stimulating digestion and moving the contents of the stomach into the intestines. In these cases, Pill Curing is especially effective. Another possible cause of acute indigestion is eating while under stress: The liver becomes hyperactive and impairs the digestive function of the spleen. Treatment involves soothing the liver while simultaneously stimulating digestion, and an appropriate remedy is Shu Gan Wan.

Chronic weak digestion is commonly due to a deficiency of qi or yang in the spleen, the principal organ of digestion in traditional Chinese medicine. When the qi of the spleen is deficient, it is unable to perform its functions of digestion. In addition to the typical qi deficiency signs of fatigue and pale face and tongue, symptoms of chronic weak digestion include poor appetite, weight loss, fullness and sleepiness after eating, and loose stools. A useful remedy for this condition is Six Gentlemen Teapills, since it contains herbs that relieve indigestion along with herbs that strengthen spleen qi. If spleen yang is also deficient, all the same symptoms are present with the addition of cold hands and feet, a desire for warm food and drinks, abdominal pain and discomfort after eating cold foods, and diarrhea with undigested food in the stools. In this case, the above patent formula should be taken along with strong ginger tea. The diet should consist primarily of soups and cooked foods but no cold or raw foods. Moxibustion to Stomach 36 and points on the abdomen also boosts the qi and yang of the spleen, gradually increasing the body's digestive strength.

Acute cases of indigestion are quite easy to treat, usually responding to one acupuncture treatment or a tube of Pill Curing. Chronic cases of indigestion due to an underlying spleen qi deficiency can take a few weeks to resolve. The classic point for all types of digestive weakness is Stomach 36, which responds equally well to moxa or acupuncture. If the person fails to change unhealthy dietary habits, the condition will be very difficult to treat.

INSOMNIA

Insomnia can occur as a result of excess conditions such as liver fire, heart fire, and food stagnation. It is also a symptom of deficiency, especially heart yin, blood, or qi deficiency. Although treatment for these conditions varies, most cases respond well to variations of Emperor's Tea since it has nourishing sedatives along with herbs that clear heat. A number of effective remedies for insomnia are available in the form of patent medicines, including Emperor's Tea, An Mien Pien, and An Shen Bu Xin Wan.

When insomnia occurs, lifestyle changes also help. As bedtime approaches, avoid stimulation by turning off most of the lights and staying away from televisions or computers. Going to bed either too full or too hungry can also disturb sleep patterns. Too many sweet foods or caffeinated beverages may also cause insomnia.

Treatment options for insomnia vary greatly, depending on the severity of the condition. Certain acupuncture points have strong sedating qualities, such as points on the wrist (Heart 7) and ear, both of which are named "Spirit Gate," as well as a point between the eyebrows (Yintang). When these points are needled, the brain releases natural opiates; the patient frequently falls asleep and wakes feeling refreshed. Receiving an acupuncture treatment late in the day reduces stress and promotes restful sleep. Chronic insomnia requires herbal therapy that addresses the underlying condition, often consisting of herbs from the category of "substances that nourish the heart and calm the spirit."

MENSTRUAL PAIN

Painful menstruation can arise from causes that include emotional factors, cervical or uterine abnormalities, cysts or tumors, or endometriosis. In traditional Chinese medicine, most patterns are variations on deficiency or stagnation of qi and blood. When qi is more stagnant than blood, symptoms of premenstrual syndrome (PMS) and pain in the breasts, ribs, abdomen, and back can occur, along with a scanty menstrual flow with some clots. The treatment principle is to regulate qi, and the classic herbal formula for that is Xiao Yao Wan.

When blood is more stagnant than qi, symptoms include sharp abdominal pain that is relieved after the menstrual blood flow begins. The blood is darker than normal with dark clots. The classic formula for this pattern is Tao Hong Si Wu Tang ("Four Substance Decoction with Safflower and Peach Pit").

If the pattern is one of qi and blood deficiency, dull pain occurs after the menstrual flow is finished. The pain, which is relieved with pressure, may be accompanied by fatigue, pale face and tongue, dizziness, and a weak pulse. The standard formula to tonify qi and blood is Ba Zhen Tang ("Eight Precious Ingredients Decoction"). It is available as the patent remedy Nu Ke Ba Zhen Wan. In all cases of menstrual pain, Yan Hu Suo Zhi Tong Pian can be used along with the other herbs to help relieve the pain.

Acute menstrual pain can sometimes be relieved with just a single acupuncture treatment, depending on the severity of the underlying pattern of disharmony. If there is pain due to stagnation from cold, moxibustion also provides immediate relief. In chronic cases, it usually takes up to three months or more for the cycle to return to normal.

PREMENSTRUAL SYNDROME

Premenstrual syndrome (PMS) is a common condition that occurs in the seven to ten days before menstruation and disappears shortly after bleeding begins. Caused by fluctuations in the hormonal balance of estrogen and progesterone, its symptoms include nervousness, irritability, emotional ups and downs, depression, water retention, and sore breasts.

From the point of view of Chinese patterns of disharmony, all of these symptoms can be traced to a stagnation of liver qi. Since the liver stores the blood and regulates the smooth flow of qi, it is almost always the organ involved in menstrual problems. When liver qi flows smoothly, the menstrual cycle is also smooth. The classic herbal formula for liver qi stagnation is Xiao Yao Wan. It is taken daily until bleeding begins, discontinued until menstruation is complete, and then taken daily again. This schedule is followed for three or four months; then a break is taken for a month. If symptoms persist, another three-month course of treatment can be undertaken. This is one of the most commonly prescribed of all the Chinese traditional formulas, and many women have experienced great relief from its use. It is also appropriate for men with symptoms of liver qi stagnation such as nervousness, irritability, and depression.

Acupuncture and moxibustion therapy are also highly effective in treating PMS symptoms. Often, a patient experiences complete relief while still in the practitioner's office. A powerful point known as "Great Pouring" (Liver 3) is often needled with powerful effects. This point can also be massaged by a person experiencing PMS symptoms or simply the stress of everyday life. Although acupuncture relieves acute symptoms quickly, chronic cases usually require two or three months of weekly acupuncture and daily herbal therapy before the condition is resolved.

Dietary therapy involves avoiding sweets, strong spices, hot peppers, and stimulants, especially coffee, which heats the liver and can actually cause this condition. Avoiding stress at this time also helps balance the energy of the liver.

PROSTATITIS

Prostatitis is an inflammation of the prostate gland often due to an acute bacterial infection. A urinary tract infection often accompanies prostatitis. Prostatitis symptoms include difficulty urinating, frequent urge to urinate, and pain in the prostate area. In acute cases of prostatitis, either acupuncture or herbs can provide immediate relief, while chronic cases take longer to resolve, depending on the severity of the condition.

Conventional Western treatment is antibiotic therapy, bed rest, and consumption of adequate fluids. In Chinese medicine, treatment of this condition, which corresponds to the pattern of lower burner damp heat, is the same as in acute urinary tract infections: Ba Zheng San. An herb that is especially effective in acute prostatitis is Vaccaria seed (wang bu liu xing). It is the chief ingredient in the patent medicine Prostate Gland Pills, an effective remedy for this condition.

Chronic prostatitis is often the result of deficiency of yin, yang, or qi in the kidneys. Treatment is Rehmannia Six Teapills, to which a practitioner often adds herbs specific to the patient's constitution and complaint. If there is a deficiency of yang, warm herbs such as aconite root (fu zi) and cinnamon bark (rou gui) are added.

SCIATICA

In sciatica, pain travels from the buttocks down the back of the leg, following the course of the sciatic nerve. Sciatica is usually caused by a lower back disk injury, usually a slipped disk pressing on the nerve; it's also possible that the nerve compression is in the pelvis or buttocks. Acupuncture is exceptionally effective for this condition: Many people experience immediate relief. Points are selected along the course of the sciatic nerve. The most important points are located on the gallbladder meridian and urinary bladder meridians. If sciatic pain is due to a severe injury to a spinal disk, treatment can take months and sometimes only brings partial relief. Moxibustion is also very helpful, as long as there is no underlying heat condition. The patent medicine Sciatica Pills is also quite effective in relieving the pain and inflammation. If there is accompanying low back pain, Du Huo Ji Sheng Wan can also be taken.

SINUSITIS

This uncomfortable condition can be caused by a bacterial, fungal, or viral infection, or it can arise from an allergic reaction. Depending on the sinus cavities involved, pain occurs in the forehead, between the eyes, or in the mouth area. Typically, there is a yellow or green discharge from the nose, often dripping into the throat. In addition to the pain, the head feels heavy. The condition can become chronic, especially when a person has repeated colds. Unless a person gets sufficient rest, avoids mucus-forming foods, and recovers fully, the sinuses will not drain completely. It is important to treat this condition as early and aggressively as possible to prevent a serious infection that requires antibiotic treatment. A vicious cycle of repeated infections and antibiotic use can develop, further weakening the immune system and making the person more prone to future infections. Traditional diagnostic patterns for sinusitis are wind cold, wind heat, lung heat, or liver and gallbladder fire that has ascended to the head. While each pattern has a different treatment, herbs and acupuncture points are used in all the patterns.

Acute conditions respond to acupuncture and herbal therapy within a few days. Needling points alongside the nose, such as Large Intestine 20 and the extra points Bitong or Yintang, is exceptionally effective at clearing the nasal passages and sinuses. These points are a little painful for about a second or two, but the discomfort is usually rewarded with an immediate clearing of the nasal passages and sinuses. Other points are selected according to the specific pattern of disharmony underlying the sinus problem. A good base herbal formula for the practitioner to work from is Xanthium Powder (cang er san), which comprises *Xanthium* fruit (cang er zi), magnolia flower (xin yi hua), *Angelica dahurica* root (bai zhi), and field mint or peppermint (bo he). Since this formula is on the warm side, some cooling herbs such as honeysuckle flowers (jin yin hua) and *Scutellaria* root (huang qin) are added when signs of heat (fever or yellow mucus) are present. An appropriate patent medicine is Bi Yan Pian for the nasal and sinus congestion, along with a heat-clearing formula such as Chuan Xin Lian Antiphlogistic Pills.

Diet is especially important in any disharmony involving mucus, since many foods tend to increase it. The patient should avoid cold, greasy, and excessively spicy foods. Sweets make the condition worse, sometimes with immediate feedback from the sinuses in the form of more congestion and pain. Once an acute attack has been cleared, *Codonopsis* root (dang shen) or *Astragalus* root (huang qi), herbs that tonify the spleen, should be taken. They can be found in patents such as Shen Qi Da Bu Wan. When spleen qi is strong, less mucus is produced, and the immune system is better able to fight off the colds that lead to sinusitis.

SORE THROAT

Sore throat can be acute or chronic. Acute cases are typically due to wind heat, with accompanying symptoms of fever, possibly a cough with yellow phlegm, and a floating, rapid pulse. The classic formula for this diagnosis is Yin Qiao Jie Du Pian. The sooner it is taken once symptoms arise, the more quickly and effectively it clears the condition. If the sore throat is especially severe, add Chuan Xin Lian Antiphlogistic Pills. If the sore throat continues to get worse, seek medical attention immediately to determine if the condition is a strep infection.

Acute sore throats usually subside after a day or two of herbal therapy and acupuncture. The most commonly used points are Large Intestine 4 and Large Intestine 11 ("Crooked Pool"), located on the hand and arm. If the pain is especially severe, a point near the base of the thumb on the palm side (Lung 10) is very effective. Since this point can be painful to needle, it is usually reserved for more severe throat pain. In these cases, the patient is willing to tolerate a little discomfort from the needles in order to get relief from the throat pain.

A chronic sore throat can have yin deficiency as the underlying cause, since the lack of cooling yin can lead to chronic inflammation. Other symptoms of yin deficiency are a thin, rapid pulse, red tongue with little or no coating, dry mouth, night sweats, and irritability or insomnia. The treatment principle is to tonify yin and clear the heat with standard formulas such as Rehmannia Teapills. It might be necessary to take the formula for a few months for it to have a long-term effect.

STRESS

Modern, industrialized societies run at such a fast pace, constant stress and anxiety are often considered by many people to be normal. Many people won't even realize they're under stress until they are diagnosed with a stress-related condition such as high blood pressure or they have a stroke or heart attack. Of course, the best way to deal with stress is to eliminate as many possible sources of it as possible. Stress-reduction techniques such as qi gong, meditation, yoga, exercise, or spiritual practices can greatly lessen the effects of stress on both the mind and body.

The effects of acupuncture in reducing stress are truly remarkable. Patients always seem to be more emotionally calm after a treatment. Certain points have especially calming effects, making them effective in treating insomnia, addictions, and anxiety disorders. In some cases, a practitioner may tape a small bead to a point on the ears known as "Spirit Gate." The person can then stimulate this point by pressing on the bead, helping maintain the calming effects of the acupuncture treatment. Some patent remedies used for their calming effects are Emperor's Tea or An Mien Pien. Stronger extracts to reduce anxiety or induce sleep can also be obtained through practitioners. Zizyphus Seed Stress/Sleep Formula, a concentrated liquid extract, is very fast-acting and effective for stress or insomnia, depending on the dosage. In addition, some herbs, known as adaptogens, help the body withstand the effects of stress. These include tonifying herbs such as ginseng, *Astragalus, Codonopsis,* and reishi mushroom. Researched extensively in Russia and China, the effectiveness of these herbs as adaptogens is well documented. Some patents that contain adaptogens are Ginseng Royal Jelly Vials, Extractum Astragali, and Kwei Be Wan.

URINARY TRACT INFECTION

A urinary tract infection (UTI) may be caused by bacteria in any part of the urinary tract, including the kidneys, ureters (the tubes that carry urine to the bladder from the kidneys), urethra (the tube that empties the bladder during urination), or bladder (the sac that holds urine before it is released through the urethra). The bacteria that cause UTIs most often enter the urethra and travel up through the urinary tract. Although men can experience infections of the urinary tract, women are much more likely to get them, for a number of reasons. First, because a woman's urethra is shorter than a man's, bacteria can more easily reach the bladder. Second, expectant mothers may be at higher risk for infections of the kidneys because a fetus can put pressure on the ureters. Finally, sexual intercourse can push bacteria into the urethra. Wearing a diaphragm can put pressure on the urethra and make it harder for a woman to completely empty her bladder, causing bacteria to collect and flourish in the un-eliminated urine. The symptoms of UTI are the same for men and women: Frequent, painful urination and some difficulty when urinating. UTIs can be acute or chronic. A number of factors increase a person's risk of UTI, such as a new sexual partner, a diet high in carbohydrates and low in protein, and not drinking enough water. The underlying pattern of chronic UTIs in traditional Chinese medicine is usually kidney yin deficiency. Other symptoms include a red tongue with very little coating, irritability, and night sweats. With the cooling aspect of the kidneys depleted, the heat generated by yin deficiency can lead to a chronic inflammation. Western medicine treats UTIs with antibiotics, but unless the underlying yin deficiency is rectified, as soon as a person gets rid of one infection with antibiotics, another one sets in. This cycle can be repeated, causing other problems from the side effects of the drugs. In Chinese medicine, the standard treatment for chronic UTI is to tonify yin and clear heat with a formula such as Zhi Bai Di Huang Wan.

The most common pattern associated with an acute UTI is damp heat in the urinary bladder. Symptoms are fever, possibly chills, burning urine, pain in the back or lower abdomen, an urgent need to urinate frequently, a red tongue with a thick yellow coat in the back, and a full, slippery pulse. An infection at this stage is best treated by a practitioner, since the infection can easily become more serious and spread through the kidneys. A patent medicine that sometimes works at this stage is Long Dan Xie Gan Wan. A strong decoction using the traditional formula known as Ba Zheng San ("Eight Ingredient Powder to Correct Urinary Disturbances") is often recommended.

Acute cases often respond very quickly to acupuncture and herbs, sometimes in a few days. The most effective acupuncture point is Ren 3 ("Middle Summit"), located directly over the urinary bladder. Another important point is Spleen 9 ("Yin Tomb Spring"), located below the knee along the inside of the tibia bone. This point is often sensitive to pressure if there is a UTI, and it is very useful for all types of imbalances of the urinary tract. Its traditional functions are to transform damp stagnation and benefit the lower burner.

During therapy for UTIs, it is important to avoid sweets completely. Eat a protein source at every meal to make the urine more acidic and less hospitable to bacteria. Wear cotton underwear to ensure that air circulates and prevents a damp environment. Abstaining from sexual activity is advised, but if not feasible, both partners should shower before having intercourse to avoid further infiltration of bacteria into the urinary tract.

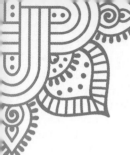

CHINESE HERBAL PATENT MEDICINES

Just as many Americans turn to over-the-counter medications for minor ailments, people in China have hundreds of herbal formulas available for a wide range of health problems. To fully explain the use of herbs and the art of herbal formulation is beyond the scope of this book. For this reason, this section describes patent medicines, which are already formulated for specific ailments and ready to take. This section introduces some of the best patent medicines for your home first-aid kit. Most of the patents come in the form of easy-to-swallow, tiny round pills (wan) or tablets (pian), plasters (gao), liquid extracts (zhi), or wine (jiu).

As is true for all types of home health care, these remedies are used to supplement professional medical care or as first-aid treatments. **In no way should they substitute for professional medical treatment**. Consult a skilled herbal practitioner before using these formulas. Remember that although herbal patents are natural, they have strong actions on the body and must be used according to specific guidelines and for specific symptoms. In the absence of a professional diagnosis or if there is any doubt about the condition, it is better to take no herbs at all rather than take the wrong ones. In most cases, the wrong patent formula will not have serious side effects, but the body can behave in unexpected ways. Follow these general guidelines for use:

- Do not exceed the recommended dose.
- Do not use during pregnancy.
- Keep out of reach of children.

Herbs can have a stronger effect on children, the elderly, or those who are debilitated, so dosages should be decreased for use by them. Children younger than 1 year should not be given herbal medicine without the advice of a practitioner experienced in pediatrics.

Take the patents with water (warm water aids assimilation). Bear in mind that patents are made with herbs, which are a type of food; so, the amount taken at one time will be larger than what you may be used to. For example, a dose of a prescription drug is usually 1 to 2 pills whereas in Chinese medicine a dose is more likely to be 8 to 12 pills.

A person with a sensitivity to one or more ingredients in a patent may develop an allergic reaction. Symptoms include skin rash, itching, difficulty breathing, diarrhea, constipation, or stomachache. If any of these symptoms occurs, discontinue use immediately. If symptoms persist, seek medical care.

The patent medicines described in the following section are grouped according to their actions. For each patent, the most commonly used name appears first. A guide to its pronunciation follows its Chinese name (within parentheses), and the English translation of the Chinese name appears last (within quotation marks). When purchasing patent medicines yourself, read labels carefully to be sure you're getting high quality herbs: Manufacturers of lesser quality herbs often copy the packaging of the reputable factories, so look for the full name of the manufacturer on the label.

FORMULAS FOR COUGHS, COLDS, FLU, ALLERGIES

BI YAN PIAN (BEE YAHN PYEN); "NOSE INFLAMMATION PILLS"

Indications: Acute or chronic nasal congestion, allergies, runny nose due to common cold

Functions: Dispels wind cold or wind heat, clears the nasal passages

Description: Bi Yan Pian is one of the more popular over-the-counter medicines. It is highly effective for nasal or sinus congestion as in the common cold, allergies, rhinitis, and sinusitis. The major herbal decongestants in this formula are magnolia flower (xin yi hua), *Angelica dahurica* (bai zhi), and *Xanthium* (cang er zi). These three herbs are effective individually, but their synergistic effect upon the nasal passages and sinuses is nothing short of remarkable. After prescribing this remedy dozens of times over the years, the only side effect one experienced practitioner has seen is some dryness in the mouth and throat. This occurred in only two cases, and it was alleviated by decreasing the dose. This example points to the need for assessing each case and prescribing an herbal remedy based on the individual's constitution. The individuals who experienced excessive dryness both had an underlying yin deficiency, which means that their body's ability to maintain a moist environment was impaired. Herbs that have a drying nature, as in this formula, tend to push that imbalance even further.

Bi Yan Pian can be used for sinus infections; it contains heat-clearing herbs such as *Phellodendron* (huang bai), forsythia (lian qiao), *Anemarrhena* (zhi mu), and wild chrysanthemum (ye ju hua). When treating an infection, it is best to be as aggressive as possible, since it can quickly progress to a more serious condition. For this reason, this patent formula is often combined with one that focuses more on clearing infections such as Chuan Xin Lian Antiphlogistic pills. In addition, when treating any infection with herbs, it is essential to begin taking the herbs as early as possible, take them regularly until the infection is gone, and then continue them for a day or two after the symptoms are gone. This last step is important because if treatment is discontinued early, it is possible to kill off enough bacteria to alleviate symptoms while still leaving enough behind to multiply again. Once an infection has been partially cleared with herbs and allowed to come back, it is much more difficult to clear it with the same herbs in a second round of treatment.

CHUAN BEI PI PA GAO (CHWAHN BAY PEE PAH GOW); "FRITILLARIA LOQUAT SYRUP"

Indications: Cough due to lung heat or dryness, with phlegm that is difficult to expectorate; a dry cough with no or little phlegm

Functions: Clears lung heat, moistens the lungs, stops coughing

Description: This soothing syrup is appropriate in cases of lung dryness that is due to wind heat, common colds, or smoking. Its chief ingredients are *Fritillaria* (bei mu) and loquat leaf (pi pa ye). Loquat leaf is especially useful for a heat-type cough, which is a cough with sticky phlegm that is difficult to expectorate. Loquat leaf comes from the same tree that produces the small delicious loquat fruits (*Eriobotrya japonica*). *Fritillaria*, the other chief ingredient, is an expectorant that is moistening to the lungs, an important action when a cough is nonproductive.

CHUAN XIN LIAN ANTIPHLOGISTIC TABLETS (CHWAHN SHIN LYAHN); "ANDROGRAPHIS ANTI- INFLAMMATORY TABLETS"

Indications: Inflammation due to excess heat, swollen glands, severe sore throat, viral infections, bacterial infections

Functions: Clears heat, clears toxins, cools the blood, reduces inflammation

Description: This powerful antibacterial and antiviral formula contains just three herbs: *Andrographis* leaf, Isatis root, and *Taraxacum* root (dandelion). The combination of these ingredients produces a pronounced cooling effect on toxic heat throughout the body. Some of the bacterial infections this patent medicine treats are acute sore throat, swollen glands, lung abscess, pneumonia, urinary tract infections, and dysentery. It can also be used for viral infections such as influenza and hepatitis.

The chief ingredient, *Andrographis paniculata* (chuan xin lian), has been shown to inhibit the *Staphylococcus*, *Streptococcus*, and *Shigella* organisms that can cause various infections. It is extremely bitter—its name in Chinese translates to "pierce the heart lotus," meaning it is so bitter, its flavor "pierces the heart." One herbalist recalls that while working in a Chinese herbal pharmacy some years ago, he noticed an extremely bitter taste in his mouth. When he turned around, he saw that a teacher had opened the drawer containing the *Andrographis*, 20 feet from where he was standing! Because of its bitterness, *Andrographis* is usually taken in pill form.

The second ingredient, *Isatis tinctoria* (ban lang gen), also has antiviral and antibacterial actions. Its broad antimicrobial effect has been shown to inhibit the bacteria that cause dysentery, salmonella, strep infection, and typhoid. *Isatis* has strong antiviral action against hepatitis and encephalitis. This is highly significant, since Western medicine has virtually no weapons against viral infections.

The third ingredient is the much-maligned dandelion (pu gong ying), a major medicine in both Western and Chinese herbalism. Traditionally used for breast abscesses, jaundice, and urinary tract infections, dandelion has impressive antibacterial effects against the pathogens that cause strep throat, pneumonia, dysentery, meningitis, diphtheria, and tuberculosis—all from a plant that is relentlessly sprayed with herbicides by the unsuspecting suburban homeowner!

CHUAN XIONG CHA TIAO WAN (CHWAHN SHUHNG CHAH TYOW WAHN); "LIGUSTICUM AND GREEN TEA PILLS"

Indications: Headache and nasal congestion due to wind cold
Functions: Relieves headache and expels wind cold
Description: This remedy is specifically indicated for a headache along with wind cold symptoms of the common cold, such as stiff neck and shoulders, nasal congestion, a desire for warmth, and a slower than normal pulse. It is meant to be taken along with green tea, which helps maximize the healing action of the other herbs. Recent research has shown that green tea also has strong antioxidant properties, meaning it helps break down free radicals, substances involved in the aging and disease processes.

The chief herb in the formula is *Ligusticum wallichii* (chuan xiong), a highly aromatic plant with strong circulatory properties. A strong analgesic (pain reliever), it relieves the headaches that occur with a cold, and it is used in many herbal formulas to direct the formula's action to the head. Another ingredient is *Notopterygium* root, a fragrant herb that releases tension in the muscles of the shoulders and neck. Since the trapezius muscles extend from the upper back to the neck and head, tightness in that muscle group can lead to an occipital headache (the back of the head at the base of the skull). The inclusion of *Angelica dahurica* root (bai zhi) has the dual function of clearing sinus and nasal congestion and relieving the pain of frontal headaches (pain in the forehead). Wild ginger (xi xin) is another analgesic herb in the formula that acts as a decongestant. Its North American relative grows in the coastal redwood forests of California; when chewed, its gingery flavor quickly numbs the tongue, demonstrating its ability to act as a local anesthetic.

Chuan Xiong Cha Tiao Wan is also useful in dizziness and loss of balance due to labyrinthitis, an inflammation of the inner ear. This patent's ability to increase circulation to the head helps facilitate healing in this ailment, for which there is no conventional treatment. Since it is very warming, this remedy should not be used for headaches due to wind heat with symptoms such as sore throat, fever, and a faster than normal pulse or headaches due to liver heat rising to the head with its symptoms of rapid pulse, red face, and anger. It should also not be used when the headache is caused by a deficiency condition such as deficient qi, deficient blood, or deficient yin.

ER CHEN WAN
(UHR CHEN WAHN);
"TWO OLD-MEDICINE PILLS"

Indications: Excessive phlegm in the lungs and stomach with nausea, cough with abundant clear mucus

Functions: Regulates qi, reduces phlegm and dampness, harmonizes the stomach

Description: The two "old medicines" referred to in the name are aged citrus peel (chen pi) and *Pinellia* tuber (ban xia). The quality of these herbs is considered to improve with age. In fact, *Pinellia* is considered toxic until it is aged and treated with ginger. Citrus peel, the other chief ingredient, is a delightful medicinal with a sweet fragrance that is especially pronounced in the high-quality aged tangerine peels. It increases secretion of gastric juices, which aids digestion; and has antibacterial effects.

This patent formula is indicated for a damp phlegm cough, which is associated with expectoration of copious amounts of clear or light-colored phlegm. In addition to their drying, expectorant activity, the two chief herbs in the formula alleviate the vomiting and nausea that sometimes accompany this condition. If the cough is due to the common cold, take this patent along with a formula such as Gan Mao Ling that helps eliminate the pathogen that caused the cold.

GAN MAO LING
(GAHN MAO LING);
"COLD FORMULA"

Indications: Cold or flu due to either wind heat or wind cold with fever, mild chills, sore throat, and stiff neck

Functions: Expels wind, clears heat, expels viruses

Description: Its extraordinary effectiveness makes Gan Mao Ling an extremely popular patent. You can use it to prevent a cold when you've been exposed to someone with a cold or to clear a cold or flu when it has already taken hold. In many cases, a few doses of Gan Mao Ling at the first sign of cold symptoms completely alleviates all symptoms, but it is also frequently all that is needed to relieve full-blown cold symptoms. It is an excellent base formula since it is effective in both cold and heat illnesses. If symptoms include nasal and sinus congestion, the formula can be taken with Bi Yan Pian. If a sore throat occurs along with the cold, it can be taken with Chuan Xin Lian Antiphlogistic Pills. If there is accompanying nausea or diarrhea, Curing Pills or Lophanthus Antifebrile (Huo Xiang Zheng Qi Wan) can be added.

MA HSING CHIH KE PIEN (MAH SHING JIH KEH PYEN); "EPHEDRA APRICOT STOP COUGH TABLETS"

Indications: Cough, bronchitis, or asthma due to heat
Functions: Clears lung heat, relieves asthma, stops cough
Description: Although this formula is used mostly to treat bronchitis with yellow phlegm due to heat, it is also quite effective in mild cases of asthma. The continual increase in the number of Americans with asthma could be due to such causes as air pollution, chemical exposure, or increased stress. Many people with asthma rely on chemical inhalers throughout the day, and some are forced to seek treatment in hospital emergency rooms on a regular basis for acute asthma attacks. Herbal medicine is quite effective in treating asthma. The results of herbal therapy range from a complete remission of the disease to a much less frequent use of inhalers.

The word ma in this formula's name refers to ma huang, or *Ephedra sinica*. This powerful herb contains ephedrine, a strong stimulant that dilates (widens) the bronchial tubes. During an asthma attack, the bronchial tubes narrow, causing a severe restriction in air flow. Inhalers open the passages to enable the person to breathe; *Ephedra* also handles the job well. When used properly, *Ephedra* is quite safe. Unfortunately, some products on the market exploit *Ephedra* as a stimulant for weight loss or recreational use, and deaths have occurred from overdoses of products that mix high levels of ephedrine and caffeine. This is a gross misuse of an important medicine. The U.S. Food and Drug Administration (FDA) is looking into the sale of these products; some states have banned products containing high levels of ephedrine. Reputable, qualified practitioners in the United States hope the irresponsible actions of some manufacturers won't cause the removal of this valuable drug from the marketplace.

Ma Hsing Chih Ke Pien can also be used for cough due to heat, with sore throat, dry loud cough, or swollen glands. When used for chronic asthma, it is best to combine it with Ping Chuan Pills, which also contain herbs that tone and strengthen the lungs. In a clinical trial in China, the bulk version of this formula was given to 40 children with asthma. All of them experienced temporary relief; out of the 19 who had chronic asthma, only two children experienced relapses up to six months later.

Warning: *Ephedra* can raise blood pressure and should not be taken by people with high blood pressure, heart disease, a history of stroke, or a sensitivity to caffeine. Some people experience insomnia if they take the remedy too close to bedtime. Do not exceed recommended dosages. Asthma is a life-threatening condition for many people. While herbal medicine can greatly help in its treatment, be sure to keep an inhaler available for emergencies, even if it seems that you no longer need it.

MINOR BUPLEURUM
XIAO CHAI HU TANG WAN
(SHOW CHEYE HOO TAHNG WAHN);
"MINOR BUPLEURUM PILLS"

Indications: Frequent colds and ear infections, colds with alternating fever and chills, malaria

Functions: Harmonizes the interior and exterior of the body, regulates the liver

Description: This patent fits easily in a number of formula categories. In Japan, where herbal formulas from China have become exceptionally popular over the past 20 years, Minor Bupleurum is the formula most frequently prescribed by medical doctors. It is used to stimulate the immune system, to treat hepatitis, and to protect against the side effects of radiation therapy. It has anti-allergy activities and is also used to treat prolonged flu and colds as well as chronic digestion problems.

Take the case of a man who had just returned from traveling in Indonesia. He was experiencing a headache and extreme weakness, with chills, fever, and sweats. From a Western diagnostic perspective, he was exhibiting all the classic signs of malaria; from the traditional Chinese point of view, he was experiencing a shao yang condition, a clear indicator for Minor Bupleurum. Since this was a serious illness, he was given the formula in the form of a decoction, three times a day. After three days, his symptoms completely disappeared. About three months later, the symptoms appeared again in a very mild form. He took the patent remedy at a dosage of 16 pills, three times a day, and the symptoms subsided again. One year later, there had been no recurrence of the malaria.

PINELLIA EXPECTORANT PILLS
QING QI HUA TAN WAN
(CHING CHEE HWAH TAHN WAHN);
"CLEAR LUNG, EXPEL PHLEGM PILLS"

Indications: Cough due to heat, with yellow or green phlegm that is difficult to expectorate

Functions: Clears lung heat, expels phlegm, stops cough

Description: This is a standard remedy for coughs due to heat phlegm, a type of cough that occurs with heat signs, especially noted by the color of the mucus. Yellow or green phlegm that is difficult to expectorate indicates a hot phlegm condition. It is essential to use cooling, moistening expectorants to dislodge the phlegm and eliminate it from the lungs, otherwise a serious infection could develop. Originally, the pathogen (the cause of the infection, or "evil qi" in traditional terminology) is often a virus. If the person's immune system fails to repel the invader, a cold or flu results. In the course of the illness, the lungs often begin secreting large amounts of mucus. If expectorants are not employed at this point, the mucus can build up in the lungs, providing a fertile feeding ground for bacteria, resulting in an opportunistic infection (an infection that results when the immune system is weakened).

If green phlegm, indicating infection, is present, Chuan Xin Lian Antiphlogistic Pills should also be taken (3 to 6 pills, three times a day). When the mucus starts getting lighter in color and the individual is able to cough it up without difficulty, the herbs are working. As in all infections, prompt qualified medical attention is essential if symptoms worsen. In addition to herbal therapy, diet is essential in cases such as this. Sweets should be avoided, as they increase phlegm production as well as feed the infection. Light vegetable soups are easy to digest and help clear mucus, assisting the herbal formula. Do not use Pinellia Expectorant Pills for coughs due to wind cold.

YIN QIAO JIE DU PIAN
(YIN CHOW JYEH DOO PYEN);
"HONEYSUCKLE AND FORSYTHIA
CLEAR-TOXIN TABLETS"

Indications: Acute symptoms of wind heat—sore throat, fever, headache

Functions: Expels wind heat, clears heat and toxins

Description: Along with Gan Mao Ling, this is one of the most popular Chinese patent medicines. It is highly effective in clearing wind heat types of cold or flu, for which sore throat is the cardinal symptom. Other symptoms could be fever, intolerance for wind and cold temperatures, headache, thirst, and cough. Although most effective when taken at the onset of symptoms, this formula can also be taken during full-blown flu symptoms. Yin Qiao Jie Du Pian can also be used for pneumonia, bronchitis, tonsillitis, measles, mumps, and inner ear infections.

Classical formulas often have their chief ingredients as part of their name. The word yin, meaning silver, comes from the Chinese name for honeysuckle (jin yin hua, or gold and silver flower). The word Qiao comes from the Chinese name for forsythia (lian qiao). Honeysuckle and forsythia are often used together due to their synergistic antimicrobial effect. Clinical research shows that honeysuckle flowers and forsythia fruit inhibit the bacteria that cause pneumonia, strep throat, staphylococcal infections, salmonella, and tuberculosis. They have both been used tradition ally for thousands of years to clear fire toxins, which include a hot, painful, swollen throat; boils; fevers; and urinary tract infections.

Another ingredient in Yin Qiao is *Schizonepeta* flowers (jing jie). The profuse purple flower spikes are highly aromatic, giving the herb a dispersing quality. When the body is first attacked by a pathogen, the most effective way to repel the invader is through the use of aromatic herbs that disperse their energy to the exterior of the body. The highly volatile essential oils open up the pores in the skin and act as a diaphoretic (induces sweating). If the pathogen has not penetrated to the interior of the body, this dispersing effect drives the pathogen out. Although it is warm by nature, *Schizonepeta* is effective in heat conditions when it is combined with cold herbs, as it is in this formula.

ZHONG GAN LING
(JUNG GAHN LING);
"SERIOUS COLD REMEDY"

Indications: Wind heat flu-like symptoms—high fever, sore throat
Functions: Expels wind heat, clears heat and toxins
Description: Although similar to Gan Mao Ling, Zhong Gan Ling focuses more on heat conditions. It contains gypsum (shi gao), a mineral used to clear high fevers, and *Isatis* (ban lang gen), a powerful antibacterial and antiviral herb, which has proved effective in treating influenza, pneumonia, meningitis, mumps, and swollen, painful throat.

Another ingredient in the formula is *Pueraria* root (ge gen), commonly known as kudzu. (This root is often used in Asian cooking as a thickening agent in sauces.) As a component of Zhong Gan Ling, kudzu has the effect of relaxing tight stiff muscles in the neck and shoulders, a common symptom of external conditions. (As a side note, recent research has shown that an extract of kudzu reduces cravings for alcohol, helping alcoholics to reduce their consumption of alcohol by 50 percent.) It is synergistic with *Notopterygium* (qiang huo), another ingredient that is effective in relieving pain in the upper body due to colds or flu.

FORMULAS FOR THE DIGESTIVE SYSTEM

HUANG LIAN SU PIAN
(HWAHNG LYAN SOO PYEN);
"COPTIS EXTRACT TABLETS"

Indications: Diarrhea, infections, or dysentery due to damp heat; frequent bloody or watery stools with abdominal pain accompanied by vomiting and fever

Functions: Decreases inflammation, clears damp heat and fire toxins

Description: This formula is essential for travel to areas of the world with primitive sanitation or questionable water quality. It is remarkably effective in killing the pathogens that cause the dreaded traveler's diarrhea.

The extract is prepared from the rhizome of *Coptis chinensis* (huang lian), and the active ingredient is berberine, a powerful constituent with strong antibiotic effects. Also found in North American goldenseal and Oregon grape, berberine gives these pills their beautiful golden color.

Huang Lian Su has strong effects, inhibiting the bacteria that cause strep throat, pneumonia, and dysentery. Studies conducted in China have shown it is as effective as sulfa drugs in treating dysentery, without their serious side effects. Clinical trials have also proved it effective in treating influenza, pertussis, typhoid, tuberculosis, scarlet fever, and diphtheria. As this list of conditions illustrates, Chinese herbal medicine is highly developed and is used by practitioners to treat serious disease as well as minor ailments. This formula should not be used for diarrhea due to deficient cold conditions.

HUO XIANG ZHENG QI WAN
(HAW SHAHNG JUNG CHEE WAHN),
LOPHANTHUS ANTIFEBRILE;
"AGASTACHE QI NORMALIZING PILLS"

Indications: Summer damp stomach flu, with nausea, vomiting, diarrhea, sticky stools

Functions: Regulates the digestion, eliminates dampness, repels wind

Description: The chief ingredient in this formula is *Agastache* (huo xiang), also known as patchouli. This highly aromatic, easy-to-grow plant is in the category known as "aromatic herbs that transform dampness." The specific action of herbs in this category is to wake up the spleen with their strong aroma and eliminate dampness in that organ. Dampness in the spleen is characterized by symptoms of nausea, vomiting, fullness in the abdominal area, lack of appetite or thirst, and diarrhea. These symptoms usually arise as a result of acute gastroenteritis—what we often call stomach "flu"—which is effectively treated with this formula.

Highly effective, this formula often relieves symptoms with just one dose. This patent should not be taken alone in the case of fever, since it is warm by nature. When there are heat signs, such as fever, it can be taken along with Gan Mao Ling, Zhong Gan Ling, or Yin Qiao Jie Du Pien. It is best to take it for an additional day after symptoms subside to give digestive function a chance to return to normal.

MU XIANG SHUN QI WAN
(MOO SHAHNG SHUHN CHEE WAHN); "SAUSSUREA QI-REGULATING PILLS"

Indications: Food stagnation, indigestion, diarrhea, and flatulence

Functions: Regulates stagnant qi in the digestive organs, relieves pain in the stomach and intestines, disperses food stagnation

Description: This formula is especially effective for traveler's diarrhea and gastrointestinal discomfort when used along with Huang Lian Su. The two formulas have a powerful synergistic effect (they enhance the action of the other): The berberine in Huang Lian Su kills the pathogens that cause the digestive problem, while the carminative herbs (which relieve gas and bowel pain) in Mu Xiang Shun Qi Wan restore normal digestive function. Even in simple cases of gas or fullness, such as after eating too much or too fast, Mu Xiang Shun Qi Wan can be quite effective.

The chief ingredient in Mu Xiang Shun Qi Wan is *Saussurea lappa*, also known as *Aucklandia lappa*. This herb is very aromatic due to its high content of volatile oils, giving rise to its name, mu xiang, meaning fragrant wood. Normal function of the digestive organs requires a smooth flow of qi; stagnation of qi results in pain, distention, and abnormal activity in the organ. *Saussurea* helps promote the flow of vital energy both in the stomach and the intestines, thereby relieving pain and distention and stopping diarrhea. It acts as an antispasmodic to smooth muscle, thereby relaxing the intestines, and it inhibits the bacteria that cause dysentery. This preparation has other positive effects in the stomach as well: It contains ginger to relieve nausea and vomiting, radish seed and hawthorn berry to move stagnant food out of the stomach, and citrus peel and barley sprouts to strengthen stomach function.

PEACH KERNEL PILLS
RUN CHANG WAN
(RUHN CHAHNG WAHN); "MOISTEN INTESTINES PILLS"

Indications: Constipation due to excess heat

Functions: Lubricates the intestines, promotes bowel movement, purges heat from the intestines

Description: Peach Kernel Pills act as a mild laxative, working both as an intestinal lubricant and a purgative to the large intestine when constipation due to dryness occurs. *Cannabis* seeds (huo ma ren), peach pits (tao ren), *Cistanche* (rou cong rong), and *Angelica sinensis* (dang gui) all act to lubricate the intestine, while rhubarb root (da huang) is a purgative. Therefore, this formula is best for constipation due to internal heat or dryness associated with small, hard, and difficult-to-expel stools or a burning sensation. It's important to remember that a proper diet is the key to the prevention of constipation: A person with this type of constipation should drink sufficient water and consume high fiber foods.

PILL CURING
KANG NING WAN
(KAHN NING WAHN);
"HEALTHY QUIET PILLS"

Indications: Disorders of the stomach, such as nausea, vomiting, fullness, acidity, motion sickness, or acid regurgitation

Functions: Regulates the digestion, calms the stomach

Description: Another very popular remedy both in China and the United States and a must for every medicine cabinet, travel kit, and purse, Pill Curing is a highly effective patent medicine. Its action centers on the stomach, where it quickly alleviates nausea, vomiting, belching, excessive stomach acid, and low appetite. It can be taken 30 to 60 minutes before travel in order to avoid motion sickness.

SHEN LING BAI ZHU PIAN
(SHEN LING BUY ZHOO PYEN);
"CODONOPSIS, PORIA,
AND ATRACTYLODES PILLS"

Indications: Digestive problems due to deficient spleen, such as loose stools, bloating, weak digestion, and belching

Functions: Tonifies spleen qi, clears dampness, harmonizes digestion

Description: Shen Ling Bai Zhu Pian is a reliable treatment for chronic diarrhea or loose stools associated with qi deficiency. In such a pattern, the digestive dysfunction is due to internal weakness, not an infection from a virus, bacterium, or parasite. Typically, the symptoms develop over an extended period and appear as indigestion, poor appetite, loose stools or diarrhea, fatigue, and a pale face. All are classic signs of spleen qi deficiency, an impairment of the body's ability to digest and absorb food. For this reason, the components of the patent either strengthen digestive function and vitality or act as an astringent to the intestines. Drawing fluids out of the colon helps make stools more firm.

This formula derives its name from three major ingredients: Shen refers to dang shen (*Codonopsis pilosula*), a tonic herb often used as an inexpensive substitute for ginseng. In addition to improving digestion, many herbs that tonify qi also act to fortify the immune system. In other words, these herbs build up the immune system to prevent illness. Dang shen helps the body fight off invading pathogens that threaten the immune system. It has also shown an ability to increase the production of both red and white blood cells, which is especially significant for chemotherapy patients. Chemotherapy destroys some disease-fighting white blood cells in addition to cancer cells, reducing the body's ability to fight off disease. Chemotherapy often causes diarrhea and other digestive system symptoms as well. The word Ling in the name refers to fu ling (*Poria cocos*), a wild fungus that grows around the roots of pine trees. It strengthens the spleen and harmonizes the digestive organs, assisting in fluid metabolism and promoting immune function. The words Bai Zhu refer to *Atractylodes macrocephala*, which is an aromatic tonic that strengthens spleen qi (the qi of digestion) and dries the damp gastrointestinal environment that leads to diarrhea. This herb also increases endurance and immune function.

SHU GAN WAN
(SHOO GAHN WAHN);
"SOOTHE LIVER PILL"

Indications: Digestive disorders associated with liver imbalances, which become worse under stress; symptoms include abdominal distention and pain, nausea, belching, poor appetite, gas, and loose stools

Functions: Regulates the liver, relieves stagnation, improves digestion, relieves pain

Description: This formula is used in the condition colorfully known as "liver attacking the spleen." In this pattern, the liver is not properly functioning to allow for the smooth flow of qi. This imbalance transfers to the digestive organs, bringing on such symptoms as gas, belching, abdominal pain, indigestion, poor appetite, or loose stools. Typically, symptoms become worse when the person experiences stress. In addition to herbs that improve digestion and relieve pain and fullness, this formula contains *Bupleurum* root (chai hu), a major herb for clearing stagnation of liver function. In this way, the formula treats both the symptoms and the underlying imbalance that causes the disorder.

SIX GENTLEMEN TEAPILLS,
XIANG SHA LIU JUN WAN
(SHAHNG SHAH LOO JUHN WAHN),
APLOTAXIS AMOMUM PILLS;
"SAUSSUREA AND CARDAMON
SIX GENTLEMEN PILL"

Indications: Weak digestion due to spleen qi deficiency, with symptoms of poor appetite, nausea, vomiting, belching, and chronic diarrhea

Functions: Tonifies spleen qi, reduces phlegm and dampness

Description: A modern patent based on an ancient remedy, the classical formula Xiang Sha Liu Jun Zi Tang combines a qi tonic with digestive herbs. The tonic aspect of the formula consists of four herbs known as the Four Gentle-men: ginseng (ren shen), *Atractylodes* (bai zhu), *Poria* (fu ling), and Chinese licorice (zhi gan cao). These herbs make up the base of numerous formulas that treat deficiency of qi in the lungs and spleen with such chronic symptoms as fatigue, shortness of breath, pale face, lack of appetite, indigestion, and loose stools. The addition of citrus peel (chen pi) and *Pinellia* rhizome (ban xia) creates Six Gentlemen, a formula more appropriate for treating more acute cases of digestive imbalances with nausea, vomiting, and distention. The addition of *Saussurea* (mu xiang) and cardamon (sha ren) further increases the formula's ability to rectify digestive weakness. It is especially appropriate for people who are pale, weak, and qi deficient with accompanying digestive weakness.

FORMULAS FOR GYNECOLOGIC DISORDERS

CHIEN CHIN CHIH TAI WAN (CHYEN CHIN CHIH TIE WAHN); "THOUSAND GOLD PIECE LEUKORRHEA PILLS"

Indications: Leukorrhea (vaginal discharge)
Functions: Acts as an astringent, regulates qi, regulates blood, clears dampness
Description: This patent formula treats vaginal discharges effectively, espe-cially in cases in which the woman has a qi deficiency marked by an over-all lack of energy and vitality. It can be used for vaginal discharges, such as *Trichomonas* or yeast infections, especially when the discharge is light-colored. The ingredients have multiple functions: They clear the pathogen, act as an astringent to the discharge, and relieve pain.

XIAO YAO WAN (SHAOW YAOW WAHN); "FREE AND EASY WANDERER PILLS"

Indications: Liver qi stagnation, with irritability and menstrual imbalances
Functions: Moves stagnant liver qi; tonifies blood
Description: This classic formula could have been placed in a number of categories: It is tonifying (strengthens digestion and builds blood) and harmo-nizing (relieves irritability and harmonizes energy flow), and it regulates the menstrual cycle. It is by far one of the most popular patent remedies used in North America. Our high-stress lifestyle often leads to the disorder for which this formula is indicated: stagnation of qi in the liver. In traditional Chinese medicine, the liver governs the smooth flow of qi in the body and is impor-tant in regulating the menstrual cycle and emotional balance. If qi is stagnant, changes in the cycle and symptoms of premenstrual syndrome occur.

Xiao Yao Wan is especially useful in cases of menstrual irregularity and discomfort as well as premenstrual syndrome and its symptoms of moodiness, breast distention, and cramping. It is most effective when used for two or three months, with a one month break afterward, then another two to three months. It should be discontinued during menstrual bleeding.

The chief herb in the formula is *Bupleurum* root (chai hu), a very important plant in Chinese medicine. *Bupleurum* is well-known for its ability to stimulate the immune system, suppress flu viruses, and bring down fevers. It is also anti-inflammatory and has a tranquilizing effect. It is the chief herb for treating disorders of the liver, especially when stagnant qi leads to emotional irritability.

YU DAI WAN
(YOO DYE WAHN);
"HEAL LEUKORRHEA PILLS"

Indications: Leukorrhea (vaginal discharge) due to damp heat
Functions: Clears damp heat in the lower burner
Description: Yu Dai Wan is another effective treatment for vaginal discharge. Unlike Chien Chin, which is appropriate for both heat and cold conditions, Yu Dai Wan is specific for discharges due to heat. The main indicator for a heat-type discharge is a yellow or dark color with a strong smell. This is considered a condition of damp heat: The discharge is a form of dampness, and the yellow color and strong smell are signs of heat. Therefore, the treatment principle is to drain the dampness and clear the heat. This is accomplished through the cold, astringent action of the formula's chief herb, *Ailanthus altissima* (chun pi). The cold nature of the herb helps clear the heat, while its astringent action helps dry the discharge. In addition to nourishing herbs that assist the body's "cooling system" (yin), the formula also contains *Phellodendron* bark (huang bai), a powerful antibiotic herb that has shown great success in treating vaginitis and cervicitis from trichomonas infections. Warning: Do not confuse this herb with the philodendron, a common, poisonous houseplant.

FORMULAS FOR PAIN AND INJURIES

CHIN KOO TIEH SHANG WAN
(CHIN KOO DYEH SHAHNG WAHN);
"MUSCLES AND BONES INJURY PILL"

Indications: Traumatic injuries, bruises, sprains, and swelling
Functions: Moves blood, reduces swelling and internal bleeding, relieves pain
Description: Chin Koo Tieh Shang Wan is useful for traumatic injuries that have bruising and swelling as the primary symptoms. The chief herb in the formula is *Panax pseudoginseng* (san qi), which is also the active ingredient in

Yunnan Pai Yao. Chin Koo also contains myrrh (mo yao) and frankincense (ru xiang), two herbs that are commonly paired to increase circulation and reduce pain. These same herbs have also been used as incense for thousands of years. The essential oils that give them their heavenly aroma also act to stimulate blood circulation. Since traditional Chinese medicine sees stagnation of qi and blood as the major cause of pain, circulatory stimulants are the treatment of choice in traumatic injuries.

DU HUO JI SHENG WEN (DOO HWAW JEE SHUHNG WAHN); "ANGELICA LORANTHUS PILLS"

Indications: Cold, damp type pain and stiffness in the low back and knees with underlying deficiency of qi and blood
Functions: Expels wind dampness, relieves pain, tonifies the liver and kidneys
Description: This classic formula was first put into writing about 1,200 years ago. It not only relieves pain, it also strengthens any underlying deficiencies that make one susceptible to injury. The specific indications for the formula are pain in the lower back and knees accompanied by general weakness, stiffness, and a desire for warmth, especially in the areas of pain. While especially appropriate for the elderly due to its tonifying and strengthening qualities, it is useful for anybody with arthritis, chronic low back pain, or sciatica.

The formula derives its name from two of the principal ingredients, du huo (*Angelica pubescens*) and sang ji sheng (*Loranthus parasiticus*). Du huo is specific for rheumatic pain that is sensitive to cold, especially if it occurs in the lower body. Its pharmaceutical actions are anti-rheumatic, anti-inflammatory, and analgesic. Sang ji sheng has dual functions: It strengthens the liver and kidneys while subsequently nourishing the bones and tendons, and it relieves the pain of arthritis. As a "side effect," it lowers blood pressure and is useful in coronary heart disease. Other ingredients in the formula include the basic formulas to tonify both qi and blood, which assist the remedy in returning strength, vitality, and strong immune function, making it especially useful for long-term use by elderly or weakened patients.

SPECIFIC LUMBAGLIN, TE XIAO YAO TONG PIAN (TEH SHAOW YAOW TUHNG PYEN); "EFFECTIVE LOW BACK PAIN PILLS"

Indications: Lower back pain, muscle strains, sciatic pain
Functions: Expels wind dampness, relieves pain, tonifies yang
Description: This remedy is similar to Du Huo Ji Sheng Wan, but it is more specific for low back pain due to injuries. It comes in a blister pack of capsules that's great for a travel kit. It relieves low back pain quickly in all but the most stubborn cases.

YUNNAN PAI YAO
(YUHNAHN PIE YOW);
"WHITE MEDICINE FROM YUNNAN"

Indications: External and internal bleeding from a variety of causes

Functions: Controls bleeding and bruising, reduces swelling, relieves pain

Description: This patent medicine is one of the miracles of Chinese herbal medicine: Its ability to stop bleeding and reduce swelling and pain are legendary. During the war in Vietnam, dead Vietcong soldiers were often found with a small vial of Yunnan Pai Yao hanging around their necks. They sprinkled it on gunshot wounds to stop the bleeding while they waited to be evacuated for medical treatment. Its effects are so powerful, it can stop bleeding from stomach ulcers or cancer, hemophilia, and severe injuries. In case of excessive blood loss, a small red pill is included with each package to prevent the person from going into shock. The red pill should not be taken unless severe loss of blood has occurred and the person is losing consciousness. Of course, these are all serious conditions requiring immediate medical care.

Yunnan Pai Yao is remarkable in its ability to stop swelling and pain due to sports injuries and accidents. Although the exact formulation of this patent is considered a family secret, it is almost 100 percent *Panax pseudoginseng* (san qi). This herb is a close relative to Asian ginseng (*Panax ginseng*) and American ginseng (*Panax quinquefolium*). However, san qi is used primarily for injuries, while the others are used to build vitality and immunity. In more than 50 years of scientific study, Panax pseudoginseng has been shown to have significant benefits. It can decrease clotting time for blood, a significant benefit to people with clotting disorders.

Yunnan Pai Yao can also be used topically to stop bleeding. Wash the injured area thoroughly with water and apply the patent directly to the injury. Apply pressure, then bandage the area. For deeper wounds, squeeze the cut together before pouring on the powder and hold it shut for a few minutes. It is important to see a doctor immediately afterward in case the cut requires stitches.

TOPICAL FORMULAS FOR INJURIES

701 PLASTERS AND HUA TUO PLASTERS
(HWAH TWAW)

Indications: Pain from sprains, traumatic injuries, or muscular tension

Functions: Stimulates circulation, relieves pain

Description: Packaged as four adhesive squares, 701 Plasters are coated with highly aromatic herbs that assist in blood circulation and pain relief. To use, peel off the plastic backing sheet and place the plaster over the sore area. Within a few minutes, you will feel warmth in the area, which disappears a short time later. The pain-relieving effects last about 24 hours, after which you peel off the plaster and discard it. It is best to wait a few hours before applying another plaster, since some people can experience mild irritation from them.

These patches are very effective for soreness due to muscle strains or injuries; however, never apply them over skin that is broken. When using them to treat muscle tightness, especially in the upper back and shoulders where people typically store tension, it is important to apply them bilaterally, even if only one side is sore. If the patch is applied to one side only, it is very common for the pain to move to the opposite side! From the perspective of traditional Chinese medicine, this phenomenon is easily explained. Pain that comes and goes, such as muscle tension, is considered a condition of wind. By its nature, wind comes and goes unpredictably; it also can appear in different places without warning. Since the nature of the plaster is to disperse wind, it is important to ensure it does not have any place to reappear.

Hua Tuo plasters are nearly the same as 701 Plasters; the only real difference is they stick more tenaciously to the skin. For this reason, they are more appropriate for areas that flex, such as joints. Because 701 Plasters don't stick quite as well, they are ideal for hair-covered areas.

CHING WAN HUNG, JING WAN HONG (CHING WAHN HUHNG); "CAPITAL ABSOLUTE RED"

Indications: Burns of all kinds
Functions: Clears heat, relieves pain, promotes healing
Description: Without a doubt, this miracle cream has a welcome place in any first-aid kit. Its ability to heal burns quickly is almost beyond belief. It can be applied to first and second degree burns as long as there is no infection. As soon as the ointment comes in contact with the skin, the pain begins to recede. In China, it is used for burns caused by hot water or steam, chemicals, radiation, and sunburn. Apply the cream, then cover the burn with a dressing, which you should change daily. For simple first degree burns, no dressing is necessary. Be aware that this salve stains clothing.

ZHENG GU SHUI (JUHNG GOO SHWAY); "SETTING BONE LIQUID"

Indications: Traumatic injuries, bruises, sprains
Functions: Relieves blood stagnation, promotes healing, stops pain
Description: This highly effective liniment can be used for all sorts of injuries; however, its specialty is to reduce pain and promote healing of broken bones. If the skin is not broken, it can be applied topically to the area of injury to

relieve pain until the bone is set at the hospital. For sprains and sports injuries, it can be applied at any time. Similar effective liniments are Po Sum On Medicated Oil and Tieh Ta Yao Gin. If the skin is broken or burned at the site of the injury, use Wan Hua Oil, which is safe to apply in these conditions.

Caution: Do not use on open wounds. Some people experience a skin reaction from liniments; discontinue use immediately if a reaction develops. Avoid exposing the treated area to sun to avoid irritation. Wash hands thoroughly after applying. This patent is for external use only. Keep tightly closed and out of reach of children. Do not use Zheng Gu Shui near an open flame as it is flammable. This liniment stains clothing.

FARGELIN FOR PILES (HIGH STRENGTH), QIANG LI HUA ZHI LING (CHYAHNG LEE HWAH JIH LING); "EXTRA STRENGTH EFFECTIVE ELIMINATE HEMORRHOIDS"

Indications: Acute and chronic hemorrhoids
Functions: Invigorates blood, relieves pain, reduces swelling, clears heat
Description: Add this remedy to the list of remarkable Chinese medicines. People frequently report overnight relief from the pain, swelling, and bleeding of hemorrhoids. Note: bear gallbladder may be listed as one of the ingredients. Typically, this ingredient has been replaced by the gallbladder of a domestic animal, or the patent contains no animal products. Continued international pressure should ensure that the Chinese discontinue the practice of using body parts from endangered species.

LIAN QIAO BAI DU PIAN (LYAHN CHOW BYE DOO PYEN); "FORSYTHIA CLEAR TOXINS TABLETS"

Indications: Skin inflammations and infections
Functions: Clears heat and inflammation, relieves pain
Description: Lian Qiao Bai Du Pian is a useful formula for treating a wide variety of skin eruptions due to toxic heat, such as boils, skin infections, and poison oak or ivy. In all cases of skin inflammation, it is essential to make adjustments in the diet as well. One way the body eliminates irritating or unhealthy substances is through the skin. A diet that is high in irritating substances such as coffee and spicy and greasy foods, therefore, often leads to skin problems. In fact, coffee is so heating to the blood that it can be almost impossible to clear an individual's skin problems as long as he or she continues to drink it. Since this heat in the blood is a result of an internal process, it is very difficult to resolve skin eruptions or skin inflammation with the application of topical creams or ointments. However, when blood-cooling herbs are taken internally, the inflammation is dealt with at the source.

In one case, a young woman had been suffering for weeks from severe poison oak. Her thigh was swollen, stiff, and bright red; even a cortisone shot failed to relieve the symptoms. She was given a bulk herbal formula similar to Lian Qiao Bai Du Pian to drink three times a day; an external wash consisting of astringent herbs was also applied to relieve the itching and to help dry up the rash. In addition, her diet was adjusted to include cooling foods such as salads and carrot juice. After one week, her leg had returned to normal. She continued on a maintenance dose of the patent medicine for another week to make sure that the inflammation was gone, and she eliminated coffee from her diet.

Lian Qiao Bai Du Pian contains rhubarb root (da huang), which helps to clear toxic heat. It accomplishes this by increasing bowel movements. This purgative effect should be considered before taking the remedy.

LONG DAN XIE GAN WAN
(LUHNG DAHN SHYEH GAHN WAHN);
"GENTIAN CLEAR THE LIVER PILLS"

Indications: Excess heat in the liver causing conjunctivitis, urinary tract infection, prostatitis

Functions: Clears damp heat and fire from the liver and from the gallbladder

Description: This traditional formula treats a wide range of inflammatory conditions. Its actions are most easily understood when considered from the perspective of traditional Chinese disease patterns. This patent is indicated strictly for excess-type disorders rather than deficiency-type conditions. While deficiency conditions require a strengthening or tonifying of the body, in conditions of excess, the proper treatment is often to clear heat or drain dampness. Long Dan Xie Gan Wan is specific for the patterns known as excess heat or damp heat in the liver and gallbladder, with symptoms that include red eyes, headache, bitter taste in the mouth, irritability, and possible hearing loss. Other symptoms of "lower burner damp heat" are dark or cloudy urine, genital itching or swelling, vaginal discharge, and constipation.

The numerous imbalances Long Dan Xie Gan Wan is able to resolve are organized by organ system as follows:

- Eyes: acute conjunctivitis ("pink eye"), corneal ulcers, acute glaucoma, retinitis
- Ears: acute middle ear infection, acute external ear infection
- Urinary: acute urinary tract infection (kidney, bladder, or urethra)
- Reproductive: genital herpes, pelvic inflammatory disease, vaginal discharge, testicular swelling or inflammation, acute prostatitis
- Systemic: migraine, eczema, herpes zoster
- Liver and gallbladder: acute hepatitis, acute cholecystitis

Although the conditions listed above appear unrelated, they can share the same traditional Chinese diagnosis. For this reason, it is essential to treat the individual's traditional symptom patterns, not the Western disease name. Just as a single Chinese diagnostic category can manifest as numerous and widely different Western diseases, a single Western disease can also have a wide range of Chinese diagnoses, depending on an individual's symptoms and constitution.

In one memorable case in which Long Dan Xie Gan Wan was effective, a patient had severe conjunctivitis in one eye for a few weeks. She had already gone through a round of antibiotics with no resolution, and she was beginning to feel desperate. Her symptom pattern fit the diagnosis of excess heat in the liver, so she was given Long Dan Xie Gan Wan. In addition, a tea of chrysanthemum flowers (ju hua) was prescribed to reduce inflammation specifically in the eye. After one week of Chinese herbal therapy, the eye returned to normal. At this point, the condition of excess heat was cleared, and it was time to address the underlying weakness, a deficiency of liver yin. When the moistening, cooling, yin aspect of the liver is deficient, the organ tends to overheat, making it more prone to inflammation. For example, if a car engine is low on oil or water (yin) it has a tendency to overheat. Once it overheats, the first step is to let it cool down (clear excess heat). To address the cause of the overheating, oil and water are added (tonifying yin). In this way, traditional Chinese medicine is very thorough in its treatment of disease; it not only corrects the problem but resolves the cause as well.

In another case, Long Dan Xie Gan Wan was used to treat an attack of genital herpes in a young woman. As is often the case with outbreaks of the herpes virus, the young woman could sense the attack coming on before actual symptoms appeared, giving her a chance to begin treatment before the full-blown manifestation. Since the symptoms fit the pattern of damp heat in the liver meridian, she immediately began a course of Long Dan Xie Gan Wan along with acupuncture therapy. The outbreak was not only milder than usual but it went into remission very quickly compared with her previous outbreaks.

PROSTATE GLAND PILLS, QIAN LIE XIAN WAN (CHYAHN LYEH SHAHN WAHN)

Indications: Acute and chronic prostatitis, testicular pain
Functions: Clears damp heat in the lower burner, stimulates circulation, decreases inflammation
Description: As the name implies, this remedy is formulated for acute or chronic inflammation of the prostate gland. This disorder is especially common in males older than 40 years of age. Symptoms include dribbling or painful urination and pain in the testicles. The remedy is also useful for urinary tract infections and testicular inflammation. In two cases of testicular pain due

to trauma, one in a marathon runner and the other in a bicycle racer, a course of Prostate Gland Pills along with some rest from their athletic activity was all they needed. Treatment took only a week. Chronic cases of inflammation may require a longer course of treatment.

The chief herb in the formula is *Vaccaria* seed (wang bu liu xing), which is useful for painful swellings in the breasts or testicles.

FORMULAS FOR TONIFICATION AND IMMUNITY

BU ZHONG YI QI WAN (BOO JUHNG YEE CHEE WAHN), CENTRAL CHI TEA; "TONIFY THE MIDDLE, STRENGTHEN QI PILLS"

Indications: Qi deficiency, weak digestion, prolapsed organs, fatigue
Functions: Tonifies qi, regulates digestion, raises yang (pulls up prolapsed organs)
Description: An ancient formula, Bu Zhong Yi Qi Wan has a long history of resolving digestive problems and prolapsed organs, both conditions due to qi deficiency. Although primarily composed of tonifying herbs, this formula also contains two herbs that perform a task unique to Chinese medicine. *Cimicifuga* (sheng ma) and *Bupleurum* (chai hu) are used as directing herbs with an upward energy; that is, in addition to their specific medicinal effects, they can also direct the effects of an herb formula to the upper portion of the body. This upward energy can also be employed to resolve organ prolapse, a condition in which an organ, such as the uterus, bladder, or rectum, sags downward due to connective tissue weakness. The formula is also useful—when prescribed and supervised by an experienced practitioner—for the condition known in Western medicine as "incompetent uterus" in which miscarriage occurs between the third and sixth months of pregnancy due to cervical weakness. In addition to strengthening prolapsed organs, Bu Zhong Yi Qi Wan can be used for other symptoms of spleen and stomach qi deficiency, such as fatigue, abdominal bloating, sensitivity to cold, and chronic diarrhea.

EXTRACTUN ASTRAGALI, BEI QI JING (BAY CHEE JING); "ESSENCE OF NORTHERN ASTRAGALUS"

Indications: Fatigue, weak immune system
Functions: Tonifies spleen qi and lung qi
Description: Available in small one-dose vials, this remedy is a 50/50 mixture of honey and *Astragalus* root (huang qi). This perennial member of the pea

family produces a large yellow root that is highly prized in Chinese herbal medicine. It is often cooked in soup bases to provide a boost to the vital energy. A safe and effective herb, it strengthens the immune system (wei qi) by increasing production of antibodies and macrophages, cells that attack disease-causing pathogens and foreign objects in the body. It is also used to strengthen spleen qi, meaning it improves digestive function and overall vitality. It helps nourish the blood and "generate flesh," making it useful for skin ulcers that won't heal and postsurgical recovery. In China, it is routinely given to women who have undergone surgery to remove fibroid tumors from the uterus. This operation frequently leaves the uterine wall in a thin, weakened state, making future pregnancies a risk. *Astragalus* is used to help surgical patients grow new muscle tissue in the uterus before scarring sets in.

The blood-building aspect of this herb can be seen in its use after chemotherapy, a procedure that causes severe disruptions in white blood cell count. Combined in a decoction with *Ligustrum* seeds (nu zhen zi), this remedy has been found to normalize the blood count.

GINSENG ROYAL JELLY VIALS, REN SHEN FENG WANG JIANG (REN SHEN FUHNG WAHNG JYAHNG); "GINSENG AND ROYAL JELLY SYRUP"

Indications: Fatigue, poor appetite, feeling cold and weak
Functions: Tonifies qi and yang
Description: Asian ginseng is a strong tonic to several organ systems. With its warm energy, it is especially appropriate for weak, cold individuals who have both qi deficiency and yang deficiency. Symptoms of this deficiency condition include fatigue, low immunity, pale face and tongue, and feeling cold all the time. It has a significant ability to reduce fatigue and strengthen the immune system. Because of its warm nature, Asian ginseng is not recommended for individuals with high blood pressure or a high metabolism with a tendency to overheat. For these individuals, American ginseng (*Panax quinquefolium*), with its cooling, moist, yin-enhancing nature, is more appropriate.

At one time considered an exotic curiosity from Asia, ginseng products such as this are now sold all over North America. It's not uncommon to find these vials sitting at cash registers at the most unlikely of places, such as convenience or liquor stores. Although the syrup contains very little ginseng, it is still quite effective at building overall energy. For more serious tonification, a stronger extract is recommended, such as the liquid Panax Ginseng Extractum or the thick syrup, "Pure Concentrated Korean Red Ginseng Tea." To truly experience the power of ginseng, there is no substitute for boiling a whole root for an hour or two and drinking the liquid.

The amount of research conducted on the effects of ginseng is staggering. Ginseng root has been found to enhance the ability of the nervous system to adapt to stress, stabilize blood pressure in cases of shock, and have a synergistic effect with insulin, which may allow a person with diabetes to reduce the amount of insulin used to control blood sugar levels.

KWEI BE WAN, GUI PI WAN (GWAY PEE WAHN), ANGELICA LONGANA TEA; "BRING BACK THE SPLEEN PILLS"

Indications: Fatigue, palpitations, poor memory, insomnia
Functions: Tonifies spleen qi and heart blood
Description: This ancient classical formula, available in convenient pill form, treats symptoms of deficiency in both the heart and spleen. This sort of imbalance often arises as a result of excessive thinking or preoccupation and is often referred to as "student's syndrome." Symptoms of spleen qi deficiency include fatigue, poor digestion, abdominal distention, loose stools, and pale face. The ingredients used to fortify the spleen are *Codonopsis* (dang shen), *Poria* (fu ling), *Saussurea* (mu xiang), *Atractylodes* (bai zhu), licorice (gan cao), and *Astragalus* (huang qi). The symptoms of heart blood deficiency are insomnia, poor memory, restless dreaming, mental restlessness, and dizziness. These are addressed by the inclusion of *Ziziphus* seed (suan zao ren), *Polygala* (yuan zhi), *Angelica sinensis* (dang gui), and longan fruit (long yan rou). Since a deficiency of spleen qi involves an impairment of the body's ability to assimilate nutrients through digestion, it often leads to a deficiency of blood. Therefore, the qi tonic herbs synergistically assist the blood tonic herbs in enriching the heart blood, another demonstration of the subtle elegance of traditional Chinese herbal medicine.

REHMANNIA TEAPILLS, LIU WEI DI HUANG WAN (LOO WAY DEE HWAHNG WAHN), SIX FLAVOR TEA; "SIX INGREDIENT REHMANNIA PILLS"

Indications: Thirst, irritability, night sweats, insomnia, weak low back and knees
Functions: Tonifies kidney yin, clears heat from yin deficiency conditions
Description: This is the classical base formula for all conditions of yin deficiency, especially of the liver and kidneys. Yin is moist, cool, and calm, and it enriches the organs and acts as a lubricant to bodily functions. When yin is deficient, chronic dryness and inflammation can occur. Yin deficiency can be compared with running a car that is low on oil: Under normal operating conditions, the lack of lubrication causes the engine to run hotter than normal; continued operation under these conditions can lead to long-term damage.

A variety of factors can cause yin to become deficient, such as overwork, lack of sufficient rest, insufficient fluid intake, stress, an overly dry environment, and excessive sexual activity. Symptoms of liver and kidney yin deficiency include a warm sensation in the sternum, palms, and soles of the feet; red cheeks; night sweats; a feeling of heat and irritability in the afternoon and evening; sore and weak low back and knees; ringing in the ears; chronic dry mouth; thirst; a reddish tongue with little or no coating; and a thin, rapid pulse. By focusing on nourishing yin and clearing the heat from the deficiency, this formula subtly and elegantly treats this wide range of seemingly unrelated symptoms. It contains three ingredients that nourish yin and three that clear the deficiency heat. The chief tonifying herb in the formula is *Rehmannia glutinosa* (di huang). In its raw state, it has a cold energy and is used to clear heat and nourish yin, making it useful in the treatment of high fevers and thirst due to diabetes. The prepared form is treated with wine to make it more nourishing to the blood and is used to treat anemia and menstrual difficulties and as an overall tonic to the kidneys and adrenal glands.

Another important ingredient in Rehmannia Teapills is *Dioscorea,* or Chinese yam (shan yao), a tonic to the lungs, stomach, and kidneys. It also induces the production of interferon, a substance manufactured by the immune system; interferon prevents viruses from replicating without disturbing normal cell function. The third tonic herb is *Cornus officinalis,* or dogwood fruit (shan zhu yu), an astringent herb with a variety of actions: It is antiallergic, diuretic, antihypertensive, antitumor, antibacterial, and antifungal, and it increases the production of white blood cells. An astringent, it prevents further depletion of yin, preventing the excessive loss of semen, perspiration, urine, and uterine blood. Another ingredient, *Alisma plantago*, or water plantain (ze xie), a strong diuretic and antibacterial herb, lowers blood pressure, cholesterol, and blood sugar, another reason this formula is so effective in controlling diabetes. A sedating herb included in the formula is *Poria cocos* (fu ling), a diuretic herb that also has a calming effect on the body. It is one of the important herbs for stimulating the immune system; it induces interferon production and contains polysaccharides that stimulate the immune system to track down and destroy cells foreign to the body. The final herb in the formula is moutan, or tree peony root bark (mu dan pi), an aromatic agent that cools the body on a number of levels. It also lowers blood pressure and decreases body temperature.

Liu Wei Di Huang Wan is a highly sophisticated formula that is useful in a wide variety of conditions. Numerous modifications to this base formula are available for specific conditions. Some of the disorders Liu Wei Di Huang Wan treats are diabetes, tuberculosis, hyperthyroidism, nephritis, hypertension, chronic urinary tract infection, and various degenerative diseases of the eyes. With some conditions, such as tuberculosis, Western pharmaceuticals are taken along with the herbs.

Note: Many of these conditions are life-threatening. As with all of the remedies in this book, the care of a qualified physician is essential while working with the herbs.

SHEN QI DA BU WAN
(SHEN CHEE DAH BOO WAHN);
"CODONOPSIS ASTRAGALUS
GREAT TONIFYING PILL"

Indications: Weak immunity, fatigue, lack of appetite
Functions: Tonifies lung and spleen qi, strengthens immunity.
Description: Shen Qi Da Bu Wan is a tonic for qi, blood, and immune function (wei qi). It is a mixture of *Astragalus* and *Codonopsis* root. Both herbs are important tonics, and combined they make a balanced formula. They have a synergistic effect, since they both stimulate the central nervous system, lower blood pressure, stimulate the immune system, and increase the blood count.

SHOU WU CHIH
(SHOW WOO CHERH);
"POLYGONUM HE SHOU WU JUICE"

Indications: Fatigue, poor vision, general debility, premature aging
Functions: Tonifies blood and essence
Description: Shou Wu Chih is another convenient liquid tonic. The chief herb is *Polygonum multiflorum* (he shou wu), also incorrectly known as fo ti. Essentially a blood tonic, he shou wu nourishes liver and kidney essence, treating such conditions as weakness, insomnia, blurred vision, and premature graying of the hair. The herb's name is due to an old tale about its discovery. As the story goes, Mr. He was an old, gray-haired man who went off into the hills to die so he would not become a burden to his family. After a few months, he wandered back into his village looking quite healthy with a full head of black hair. When questioned about how he managed to thrive so well in the wild, he replied that he had survived by eating the roots of a wild vine, *Polygonum multiflorum*. Since then, the plant has been known as he shou wu, or "black-haired Mr. He." In addition to its nourishing quality, he shou wu has demonstrated effectiveness in lowering blood cholesterol levels and inhibiting the pathogens that cause tuberculosis and malaria.

In addition to other yin and blood tonics such as *Angelica sinensis* (dang gui) and *Rehmannia glutinosa* (shu di huang), the formula also contains small quantities of cloves (ding xiang, or "fragrant spike") and cardamon (sha ren). The inclusion of these aromatic carminative herbs makes the formula more digestible. Tonic herbs, even those meant to strengthen digestive function, are often heavy and difficult to digest. For this reason, digestive stimulants are often added to tonic formulas to prevent digestive discomfort.

TANG KWEI GIN
(DAHNG GWAY JIN);
"ANGELICA DANG GUI SYRUP"

Indications: Fatigue, anemia, scanty menses
Functions: Tonifies qi and blood, regulates menses
Description: A classic blood tonic, Tang Kwei Gin comes in a liquid form that is quite pleasant-tasting when mixed in water. When used along with Women's Precious Pills, it can raise the red blood cell count, an important action in cases of anemia or fatigue after surgery or a prolonged illness. It also strengthens digestive function, helping the body absorb nutrients from food and further assisting in the production of new blood cells.

The chief herb in the formula is *Angelica sinensis* (dang gui), a sweetly aromatic root with a wide range of actions. It has a regulatory effect on the uterus, enabling contractions to be more regular (such as in cases of delayed or weak menstruation) or relaxing the uterine muscle (such as with cramps), depending on which is needed. The formula also contains vitamin B12, which is necessary to prevent pernicious anemia.

ZHI BAI DI HUANG WAN
(JIH BYE DEE HWAHNG WAHN);
"ANEMARRHENA AND PHELLODENDRON
WITH REHMANNIA PILLS"

Indications: Hot flashes, night sweats, irritability, menopausal symptoms, all due to strong heat arising from yin deficiency
Functions: Tonifies yin and clears heat from yin deficiency conditions
Description: This variation on Liu Wei Di Huang Wan has two added ingredients: *Anemarrhena* root (zhi mu) and *Phellodendron* bark (huang bai). The addition of these two heat-clearing herbs makes the formula much colder, enhancing its ability to clear heat from deficiency of yin. This makes it more useful than the base formula, Liu Wei Di Huang Wan, when deficiency heat is the major symptom as in night sweats, hot flashes, thirst, restlessness, red cheeks, and dark urine. It is very useful in treating the symptoms of menopause, where the deficiency of yin (estrogen) leads to deficiency heat (hot flashes, night sweats, restlessness). It is also effective in treating the same symptoms in people who have developed deficiency heat signs after long-term use of thyroid replacement hormones or lithium.